ADVANCES IN COMMON EYE INFECTIONS

Edited by **Shimon Rumelt**

Advances in Common Eye Infections
http://dx.doi.org/10.5772/60585
Edited by Shimon Rumelt

Contributors

Shalini Malhotra, Maria Kazimiera Maślińska, Nancy Malla, Kapil Goyal, Carlos Alberto Pantoja-Meléndez, Herlinda Mejia-López, Víctor Manuel Bautista-De-Lucio, Mariana Ortiz-Casas, Jonatha Quevedo-Martínez, Lidia Chomicz, Jacek P. Szaflik, Marcin Padzik, Justyna Izdebska, Shimon Rumelt

Published by InTech

Janeza Trdine 9, 51000 Rijeka, Croatia

Publishing Process Manager Iva Simcic

Technical Editor SPi Global

Cover InTech Design team

First published December, 2016

Printed in Croatia

Additional hard copies can be obtained from orders@intechopen.com

Advances in Common Eye Infections, Edited by Shimon Rumelt

p. cm.

Print ISBN 978-953-51-2809-0
Online ISBN 978-953-51-2810-6

For EU product safety concerns:
IN TECH d.o.o., Prolaz Marije Krucifikse Kozulić 3, 51000 Rijeka, Croatia,
info@intechopen.com or visit our website at intechopen.com.

Meet the editor

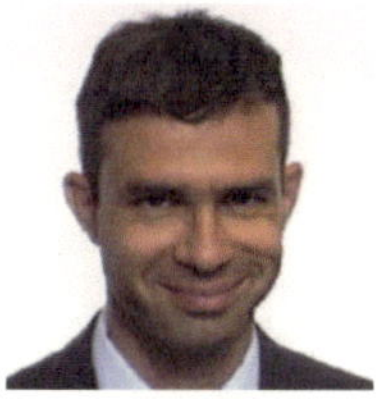

Shimon Rumelt received his medical degree and a diploma in ophthalmology from the Tel Aviv University, Israel. He completed his ophthalmology residency program at Western Galilee Medical Center in Nahariya, Israel, and then an oculoplastics fellowship at Massachusetts Eye and Ear Infirmary, Boston, Massachusetts, and vitreoretinal fellowship at Boston University. He earned a master degree in Public Administration (Health Systems) from Clark University, Worcester, MA. Shimon Rumelt is a senior ophthalmologist at the Western Galilee Medical Center, Nahariya, and is engaged with various fields in ophthalmology. He is engaged with clinical activities, surgery, research, and teaching medical students, residents, and fellows. Shimon Rumelt edited 4 books and is the author and coauthor of approximately 100 scientific articles and book chapters. He is a member of the editorial board of Evidence-Based Ophthalmology and a reviewer for multiple professional journals. He is an associate clinical professor at the Faculty of Medicine, Bar-Ilan University, Zefat, Israel.

Contents

Preface

This book is a new addition for a broad-spectrum library in ophthalmology and other specialties in medicine of "InTech." It addresses ocular infections. These infections may result in blindness if not correctly diagnosed and promptly treated. Therefore, it is essential to be fully aware and knowledgeable about the manifestations of these diseases, and this book covers some of the different aspects of them. The chapters were written by experts from around the globe and these reflect the importance of the subject.

This book gives a concise and descriptive text, including diagnostic steps, laboratory tests, and treatment options. The first chapter addresses the broad spectrum of ocular infections as an introduction for the next ones. The second chapter by Dr. Shalini Malhotra, Dr. Sharma, Dr. Bhatia, and Dr. Hans concerns with bacterial infections (endophthalmitis). Prof. Nancy Malla and Dr. Kapil Goyal discuss parasitic infections, while Prof. Lidia Chomicz specifically addresses *Acanthamoeba* infections. The last chapter on this section on specific clinical entities by Dr. Carlos Alberto Pantoja-Meléndez is on mixed ocular infections (coinfections). The last chapter by Dr. Maria Malińska and Dr. Brygida Kwiatkowska on miscellaneous issues deals with dry eyes as a factor contributing to ocular infections. This book is a balanced result of efforts to publish in timely manner and efforts to cover the topic as much as possible. Hopefully, additional books will cover more aspects of ophthalmology.

My deep gratitude is for each author for his or her time and effort. Deep appreciation goes to Ms. Iva Simcic, the Publishing Process Manager, for her extensive work to publish this book and to the publisher for an excellent project. My gratitude is for the readers for applying the material in this book to better assist patients worldwide without any limitation or barrier.

Shimon Rumelt, MD, MPA
Western Galilee Medical Center, Nahariya
Faculty of Medicine, Bar-Ilan University, Zefat
Israel

Section 1

Introduction to Ocular Infections

Chapter 1

Overview of Common and Less Common Ocular Infections

Shimon Rumelt

Additional information is available at the end of the chapter

http://dx.doi.org/10.5772/65957

Abstract

Infection may occur in any tissue of the eye, orbit, and adnexa. Infection may spread directly through contact and indirectly through blood vessels (especially valveness veins) and nerves. A proper treatment for ocular infections is imperative because it dictates the prognosis. Ocular infections may share identical clinical finding and be caused by different etiologic agents. To obtain the best outcome, a systematic approach for ocular infections is essential. This chapter describes the characteristic clinical features and manifestations of some common ocular infections and the differentiation between them and inflammations and other diseases even without using new imaging modalities such as confocal electron microscopy, anterior segment optical coherence tomography, and laboratory tests including polymeraze chain reaction.

Keywords: diagnosis, treatment, eyelid infections, conjunctiva, cornea, uvea, endophthalmitis, panophthalmitis, intraocular, retina, orbita

1. Introduction

A proper treatment for ocular infections is imperative because it dictates the prognosis. To obtain the best outcome, a systematic approach for ocular infections is essential. This chapter is aimed to describe the characteristic clinical features and manifestations of some common ocular infections and the differentiation between them and inflammations and other diseases even without using new imaging modalities such as confocal electron microscopy and anterior segment optical coherence tomography and laboratory tests including polymerase chain reaction.

Identifying and treating ocular infections can be challenging. Ocular infections may share identical clinical result and be caused by different etiologic agents. The infection is usually named according to the ocular structures involved with the suffix "itis" meaning infectious or noninfectious inflammation.

2. Eyelid infections

Infections of the eyelid include external and internal hordeolum [1]. The first one is abscess localized in the anterior lamella of the eyelid (orbicularis), whereas the internal is located in the posterior lamella (tarsus). Pain and swelling, redness, local tenderness and warmth of the eyelid characterize both. The swelling is well localized. When it is more diffuse, secondary preseptal cellulitis exists.

Preseptal cellulitis is diffuse swelling of one of the eyelids or both [2]. It includes the triad of tenderness (dolor), redness (color) and warmth (calor). The usual cause is eyelid abrasion by trauma. Preseptal cellulitis is distinguished from the more severe orbital cellulitis by the absence of proptosis, limitation of ocular movements and involvement of the optic disc (swelling) because the infection is confined anteriorly by the orbital septum.

Primary herpes simplex infection is characterized by small vesicle on the eyelid that may be accompanied by conjunctival hyperemia [3]. Necrotizing fasciitis is a rapidly progressive infection of the subcutaneous soft tissues that spreads through the fascia and may involve the eyelid and the orbit [4]. The first sign is skin erythema that spreads quickly and changes its color to purple. Later, the skin and subcutaneous tissues may separate from the deep tissues. The patient becomes toxic and suffers of severe local pain. It may be idiopathic or appear after trivial trauma or surgery. The most common causative agents are A streptococci, clostridium (with gas gangrene) and polymicrobial. Since the disease is fatal, early detection and treatment are essential.

Blepharitis is an bilateral inflammation of the eyelid margins that may be caused by infective agents (**Figure 1**) [5]. Seborrheic blepharitis causes scales over the eyelids and may accompany seborrhea. Staphylococcal blepharitis is clinically characterized by collarettes around the eyelash bases that move along the hair shaft as it grows. It is caused by staphylococcal species. Demodex blepharitis is characterized by sleeves along the base of the lash shaft and is caused by *Demodex folliculorum*. The eyelid margins may be erythematous. Patients may complain for ocular irritation, burning sensation, dryness or bouts of dryness and tearing. They may complain of stickiness or ocular tiredness/tense. Blepharitis may be accompanied by conjunctivitis (i.e. blepharoconjunctivitis) and in this case the eyelid margins show identical signs to blepharitis but the conjunctiva is also inflamed.

Phthiriasis palpebrarum is an infestation of the eyelid margins caused by *Phthirus pubis* [6]. Eggs and adults are found near the base of the eyelashes. Patients may complain from irritation. They are usually from nursery homes and the disease is sexually transmitted.

http://dx.doi.org/10.5772/65957

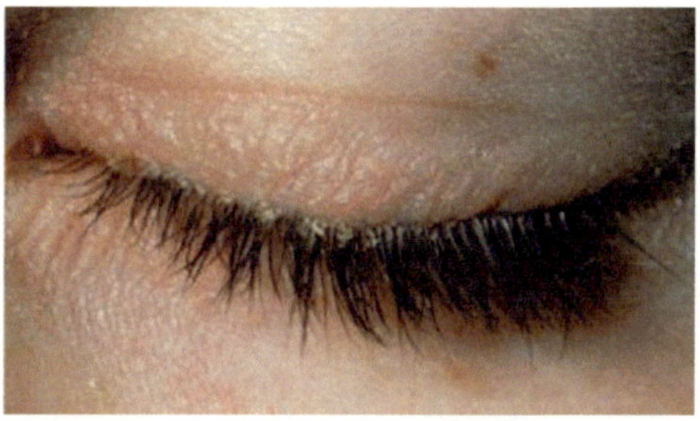

Figure 1. Blepharitis. Note the scales at the base of the eyelashes.

Treatment for localized infection such as hordeolum include warm dry compresses 3–4 times a day for 10 min each and antibiotic ointment until complete resolution is achieved or drainage, if possible. Preseptal cellulitis is treated by antibiotics such as amoxicillin trihydrate 875 mg with clavulanic acid 125 mg (Augmentin®) bid or ceftazidime 1 g/day PO or IV for a week.

Blepharitis can be prevented by eyelid hygiene. Blepharitis is treated by warm dry compresses followed by massage with tetracycline ointment for staphylococcal and seborrhea forms and fusidic acid (Fucithalmic®) for demodex. Topical azithromycin 1% is also very effective. In refractory cases, systemic antibiotics from the tetracycline family such as doxycycline 100 mg 1qd, tetracycline 250 mg qid or azithromycin 200 mg/day PO is added. Terpinen-4-ol, the main component of the essential oil of *Melaleuca alternifolia* (tea tree oil) has been demonstrated for Demodex. Blepharoconjunctivitis is treated similarly with an additional mild topical corticosteroid (such as fluorometholone (FML®) 0/1% qid or loteprednol (Lotemax®) 0.5% qid) for limited period or tear substitutes. Phthiriasis palpebrarum is treated by manual removal of all the mites and ova and treatment of the pubis with yellow mercuric oxide 1%. Necrotizing fasciitis is treated under hospitalization usually in intensive care unit. Treatment includes intravenous penicillin V 500 mg bid or intramuscular benzathine penicillin G 1.2 million units qid, aminoglycoside (e,g., gentamicin 1-1.5mg/kg/day IV tid) and clindamycin 600 mg IV tid in combination with surgical debridement and hyperbaric oxygen. patients that are allergic to penicillin receive either vancomycin 1 g bid and aztreonam 1 g tid with clindamycin instead of penicillin.

3. Conjunctival infections

Conjunctival infections manifested as conjunctival hyperemia [7, 8] (**Figure 2**). Lower eyelid follicles may accompany conjunctivitis. Discharge and preauricular lymphadenopathy may accompany be also present.

Acute conjunctivitis is less than 4 weeks, otherwise it is considered as chronic. Several entities should be mentioned. When conjunctivitis is accompanied by throat pain, fever and malaise, it is suggested as hay fever. When papillae and follicles in both upper and lower eyelids accompany conjunctivitis, adult inclusion conjunctivitis should be suspected. This is a sexually transmitted disease and both mates should be treated. Gonorrhea conjunctivitis is characterized by copious purulent discharge while other agents cause mucopurulent, mucoid or serous discharge. A form of viral conjunctivitis is hemorrhagic conjunctivitis in which conjunctival hyperemia is accompanied by subconjunctival hemorrhages.

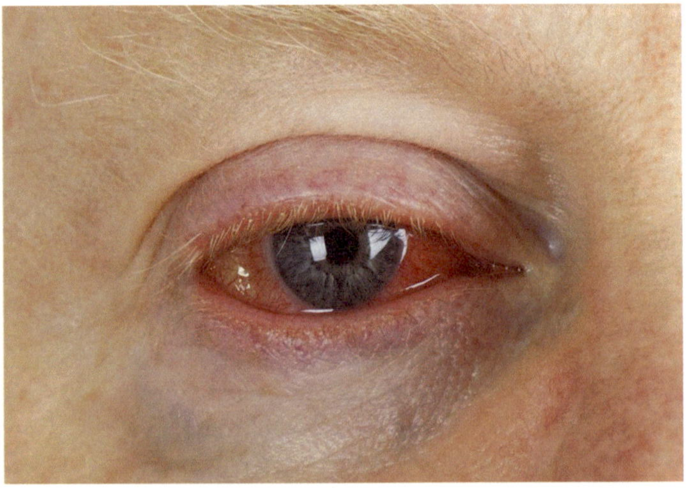

Figure 2. Viral conjunctivitis. Note the conjunctival congestion without corneal or intraocular involvement.

Conjunctival myiasis is conjunctival infestation by larvae of different types of flies depending on the habitat [9]. The larvae are tiny white and move quickly. They cause conjunctival hyperemia and the patient complains of unilateral ocular irritation. Rarely, the larva may migrate into the lacrimal drainage system and cause obstruction.

Infectious agents include bacteria, virus and chlamydia. Most microorganisms cannot invade intact epithelium. The only exceptions are *Neisseria gonorrhoeae, Corynebacterium diphtheria, Haemophilus aegyptius* and Listeria.

Infectious conjunctivitis should be differentiated from noninfectious agents such as allergic conjunctivitis and dry eyes. In neonates occurring in the first month of life, ophthalmia neonatorum is an entity that may be caused by various microorganisms such as chlamydia and less commonly by *Neisseria gonorrhoeae*. Tetracycline 1% or erythromycin 0.5% ointment qid for 3 weeks is effective for prevention and treatment.

Most of the acute viral conjunctivitis forms are self-limited and treatment is aimed to decrease discomfort and prevent secondary infection. Topical antibiotic such as sulfacetamide 10% (Sulfacid®) qid may be applied. In G6PD and sulfa-sensitive patients, other antibiotics such as Gatifloxacin (Zymar®) bid, a quinolon, may be prescribed. It is best to defer topical corticosteroid for a week to ascertain that the conjunctivitis is not herpetic or adenoviral. If no improvement is observed after a week, topical corticosteroid such as fluorometholone (FML®) 0.1% qid may be used for 1–2 weeks in tapered dosage. Patients should be instructed to prevent eye-finger-eye contact (and other contact means) especially with adenoconjunctivitis. The disease

http://dx.doi.org/10.5772/65957

is infective between 7 and 10 days. Hay fever is treated by mild topical corticosteroids such as fluorometholone (FML®) 0.1% qid or loteprednol (Lotemax®) 0.5% and nasal decongestant. Adult inclusion conjunctivitis is treated by topical and systemic tetracycline (e.g. doxycycline hyclate 100 mg once a day or tetracycline 250 mg qid). The mate should be treated as well. Myiasis is treated by removal of all the larvae from the conjunctival sac. Instillation of topical cocaine 4% may be added before removing the larvae to decrease their movement.

4. Corneal infections

The general name for corneal infection or inflammation is keratitis. The conjunctiva is usually secondarily involved as conjunctival hyperemia. The clinical manifestations vary and include corneal ulcer, abscess and/or infiltrate [10]. Corneal ulcer is distinguished from abscess and infiltrate by its staining with fluorescein. Abscess and infiltrate do not stain. The clinical findings may overlap between different etiologies.

The diagnosis of all corneal infections is based on scrapping for direct staining with hematoxylin and eosin or Giemsa, and cultures, which should be taken routinely before commencing with empiric broad-spectrum topical antibiotics. The only exceptions for obtaining corneal scarps and cultures are a marginal (near the limbus) smaller than 3 mm width flat ulcer(s) and certain typical findings such as dendrite suggesting herpetic keratitis or bilateral multiple epithelial minute defects (epitheliopathy) suggesting adenoviral (epidemic) keratoconjunctivitis.

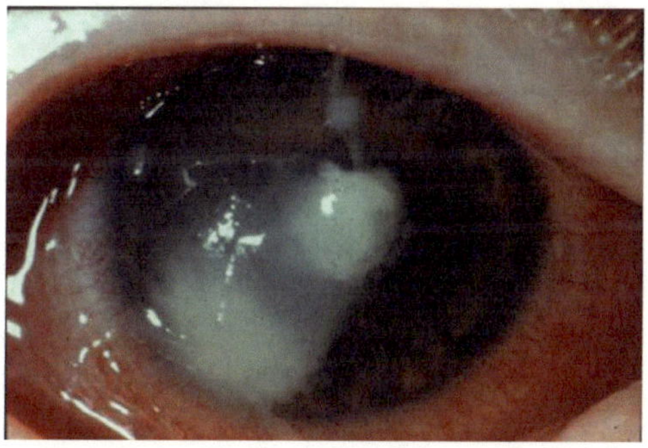

Figure 3. *Pseudomonas aeruginosa* corneal ulcer at the acute stage.

Bacterial keratitis or bacterial ulcer is usually a single solid ulcer with distinctive borders (**Figure 3**). Its size and depth may vary. It may be accompanied by an infiltrate in its base or by localized corneal edema. Infiltrate is white, more dense and distinct and is well localized in contrast to the grayish appearance and less distinctive borders of edema. A grayish, glistening appearance with secretions is a common manifestation of Pseudomonas ulcer. Flare and cells or hypopyon may accompany bacterial ulcer and they may be sterile or infected. If they appear under treatment, they indicate worsening of the infectious process. Any flare or cells in the vitreous in phakic or pseudophakic eyes indicates the development of endophthalmitis. Predisposing factors for corneal ulcer include contact lens wear, ocular trauma, dry eyes and long use of topical antibiotics and/or corticosteroids.

Herpetic keratitis a characterized by dendrites in the secondary infection. In Herpes simplex, dendrites vary in number (usually 1–3). They are coarse with widening of their ends (terminal bulbs) (**Figure 4**). Thus, they differ from Herpes zoster dendrites, which are usually numerous, small, thin and without terminal bulbs (**Figures 5, 6**). Involvement of the tip of the nose (Hutchison's sign) indicates an involvement of the eye on the same side of herpes zoster (**Figure 7**). In repeated Herpes simplex infections, the epithelial defects may form a geographic pattern and may accompanied by corneal vascularization. An important clinical test is corneal sensitivity, which is reduced in recurrent infections. Another finding is patchy sectorial atrophy of the iris that occurs mainly in the midperiphery after herpetic keratouveitis or uveitis.

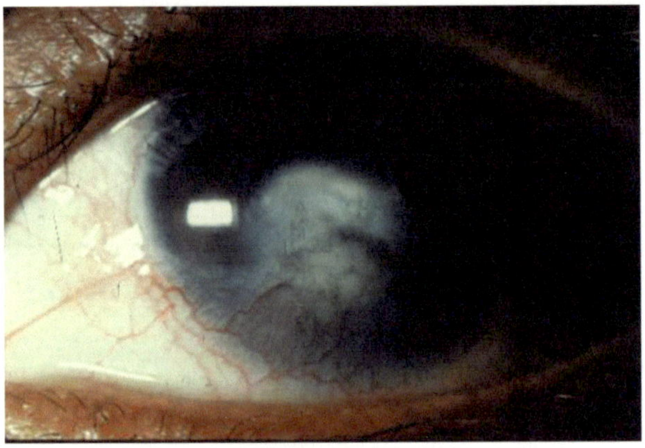

Figure 4. Corneal scar as a result of the ulcer seen in **Figure 3**.

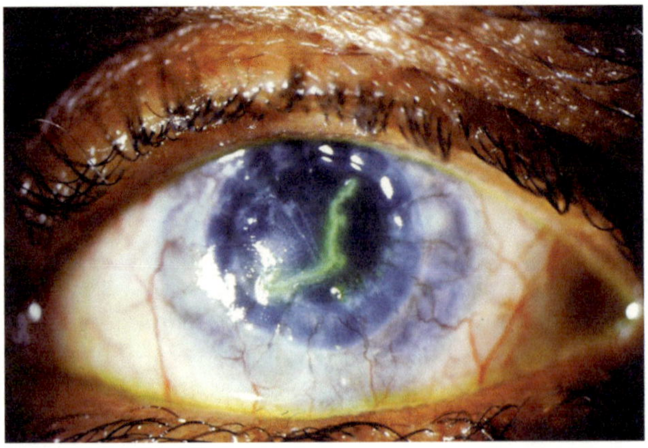

Figure 5. Recurrent herpetic keratitis with dendrite in corneal graft. The dendrite is large and has terminal bulbs.

http://dx.doi.org/10.5772/65957

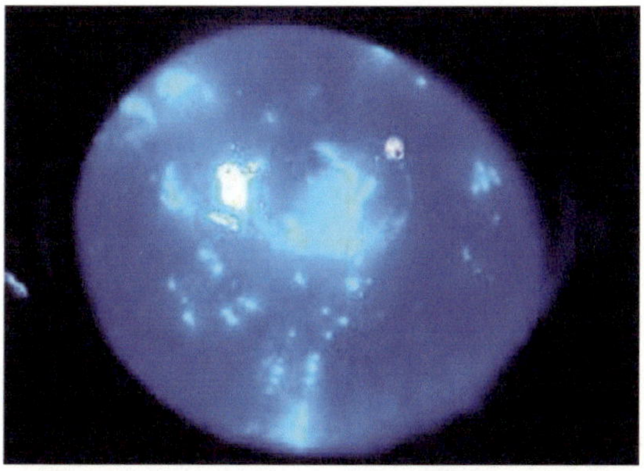

Figure 6. Corneal dendrites in herpes zoster. The dendrites are multiple and very fine. They represent immunologic reaction rather than true infection.

Fungal keratitis appears usually as multiple foci of feathery opacification of the cornea with satellites (**Figures 8** and **9**). Hyphae and yeast may be identified by confocal microscopy in the affected cornea.

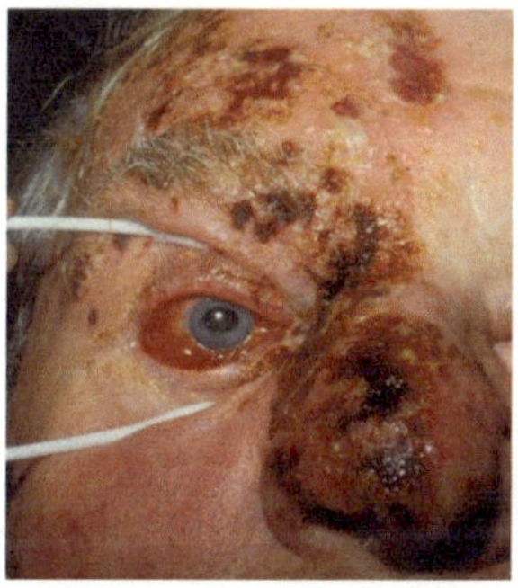

Figure 7. Herpes zoster ophthalmicus. The vesicular rash involves the dermatome innervated by the ophthalmic branch of the trigeminal nerve. Involvement of the tip of the nose indicates involvement of the eye (Hutchison's sign).

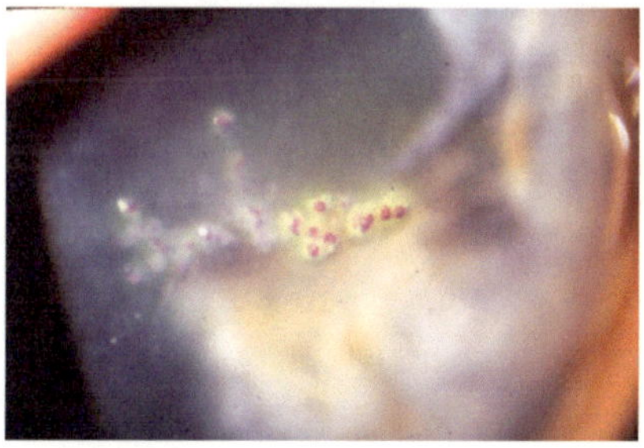

Figure 8. Fungal keratitis. Note the multiple foci.

Acanthamoeba infection may vary in presentation. The earliest clinical signs include multiple corneal epithelial cell swellings (as seen in adenoviral keratoconjunctivitis but here they are unilateral) and/or corneal edema. Late signs include perineural sheathing and stromal ring(s) (**Figure 10**). Acanthamoeba cysts may be identified by confocal microscopy. A history of contact lens wear and/or bathing in pools or sea is common and symptoms of pain are more striking than the clinical appearance. When diagnosis by cultures is impossible especially in recurrent disease, polymerase chain reaction of the involved tissue may establish the diagnosis.

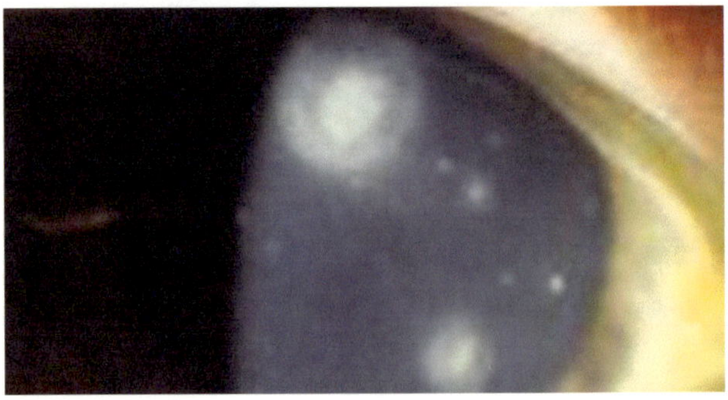

Figure 9. Fungal keratitis with multiple foci and indistinct borders.

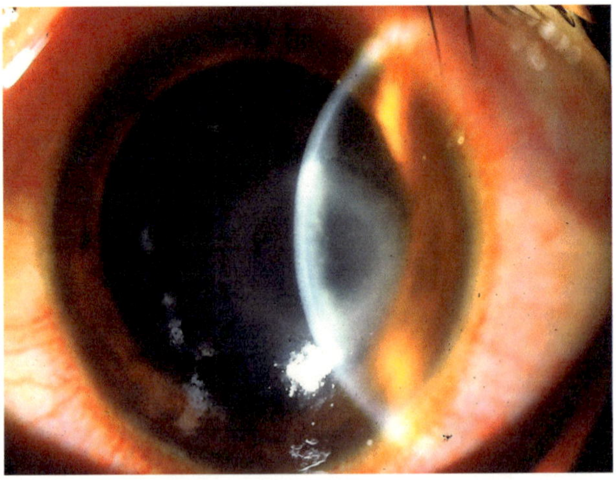

Figure 10. Immune ring in Acanthamoeba keratitis.

Corneal co-infections as other co-infections or mixed infections should be suspected when the course of the disease is atypical or when the condition deteriorates despite of treatment according to cultures and sensitivities. In such cases, repeated cultures should be obtained and broaden accordingly.

All corneal infections may result in either scarring (**Figure 10**) or melting and perforation.

http://dx.doi.org/10.5772/65957

The treatment approach differs between central and peripheral ulcers. Central ulcers are treated with topical antibiotics and are followed frequently to monitor their size and depth. Peripheral ulcers are treated with topical antibiotics and corticosteroids may be cautiously added. Treatment includes broad-spectrum topical antibiotics such as fortified cefazolin and gentamicin or moxifloxacin (Vigamox®) 0.5% every 30 min–1 h until sensitivity is obtained. Then antibiotic treatment is dictated by the sensitivity of the microorganism. In cases of pain and/or flare and cells in the anterior chamber, topical cycloplegic agent (e.g. cyclopentolate hydrochloride 1% tid) is added to decrease the pain originating from the ciliary body and/or prevention of posterior synechiae. Suspicion of infection other than bacteria should be made when no response is achieved or when the condition worsens under treatment. Additional treatment modalities include topical autologous serum, antipolymorphonuclear migration agents such as tetracycline 1% and/ or citrate 10%, which cause decrease of collagenase activity by chelating free calcium ions that are required for collagenase activity. Vitamin A (ascorbic acid) either topically 10% and/or PO (Vitamin A 500 mg bid). Liberal use of partial tarsorrhaphy is useful especially in recurrences of ulcers, exposure, dryness, corneal anesthesia or trophic ulcers and deep ones. All these means should be used in severe ulcer. Topical corticosteroids should be avoided at the acute phase of the keratitis and when the epithelium is not intact because they cause potentiation of collagenase that may lead to perforation and may also promote secondary infection. They may be used in later stage only after the epithelium healed (no corneal staining) to decrease stromal scarring. If descemetocele occurs, several surgical options exist and include anterior corneal grafts such as deep anterior lamellar keratoplasty (DALK) or non-Descemet's membrane endothelial keratoplasty (DMEK). A relatively historic treatment is placement of histoacryl for corneal perforation or descematocele. This promotes healing but also corneal vascularization, which impairs vision. Conjunctival flap (Gunderson operation) is indicated for perforation only for eyes with no potential for vision.

5. Endophthalmitis

The hallmarks of endophthalmitis are flare and white cells both in the vitreous and the anterior chamber [11]. Additional findings may include fibrin in the anterior chamber, hypopyon and retinal periphlebitis. The vision is decreased and ocular pain is noted.

Endophthalmitis is divided to two categories: exogenous (postoperative, bleb-associated and traumatic) and endogenous (source within another organ). Postoperative endophthalmitis may occur following any intraocular surgery including cataract, penetrating keratoplasty, glaucoma, vitrectomy and intraocular injections. Rarely, it may develop by spreading of keratitis or scleritis. In bleb-associated endophthalmitis, the bleb is pale and necrotic. Endophthalmitis should be suspected in any eye after penetrating keratoplasty if epithelial defect or ulcer is present near the corneal-graft interface even if there is corneal edema or signs suggesting corneal graft rejection (presence of flare and cells in the anterior chamber).

Prevention of endophthalmitis before any ocular surgery is by preparation with povidone iodide 5% that includes washing of the ocular periocular and surface. Prevention following penetrating ocular trauma injury is by intravenous broad-spectrum antibiotics (e.g. ciprofloxacin 400 mg bid) for 3 days. The data about treatment of endophthalmitis are based mainly on postoperative (cataract extraction) endophthalmitis. When endophthalmitis is suspected, vitreous samples for smears, cultures and sensitivity should be obtained before commencing antibiotic treatment. Treatment includes intravenous broad-spectrum antibiotics such as vancomycin 1 gr bid and ceftazidime 1 gr tid or moxifloxacin 400 mg/day IV as well as periocular injections and topical. Topical and/or systemic corticosteroids may be added only after the regression of the endophthalmitis.

6. Intraocular infections

Intraocular infections may involve different intraocular structures. Primarily they affect the uveal tissues (choroid, ciliary body and iris), the retina and secondarily the vitreous [12, 13]. Therefore, they may be manifesting as uveitis and/or choroidal and/or retinal lesions and the differential diagnosis is from inflammation (sterile) disorders.

Uveitis may be divided either by location to anterior; intermediate (pars planitis) and posterior, by clinical features: granulomatous versus non-granulomatous and etiology: bacterial, viral, fungal, protozoan and helmintic.

Patients may complain of ocular pain, decreased vision and/or ocular redness. The clinical signs vary. In uveitis, the anterior uvea is affected and white cells and flare are encountered in the anterior and posterior chamber and in the anterior third of the vitreous (behind the lens). Keratic precipitates (inflammatory cells and debris) over the endothelium and hypopyon may exist. The precipitates may be fine as in nongranulomatous uveitis or large and coarse (mutton fat) in granulomatous uveitis. In intermediate uveitis, the pars plana may be covered by inflammatory white band and vitreous veils resembling snowballs may be found. In posterior uveitis, white cells and flare involve the posterior 2/3 of the vitreous. They may be accompanied by retinal, choroidal or chorioretinal lesions. These lesions are key element in clinical diagnosis, which may be made by the involved tissues (retina, choroid or both), location (posterior pole, peripapillary or periphery), size, color and number of lesions (**Table 1**). For definitive diagnosis, laboratory tests are usually required.

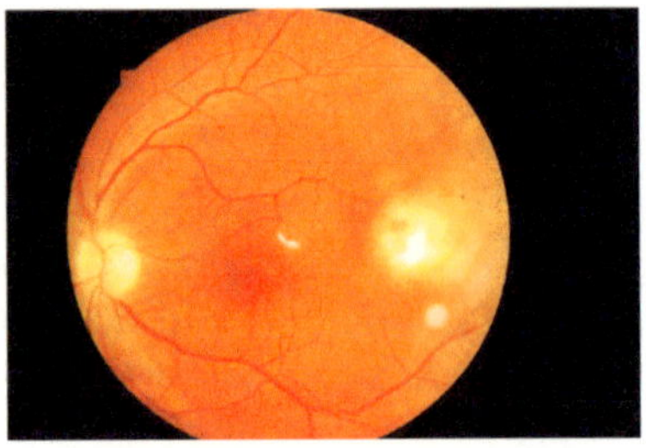

Figure 11. Toxocara retinochoroiditis. Note the active white lesion. It may appear adjacent to a chorioretinal scar.

Treatment should be first aimed at the offending microorganism. Topical and systemic antimicrobial are being used. Topical corticosteroids may be added in the absence of corneal ulcer. Systemic corticosteroids are being added if the offending microorganism is covered and the center of the macula is being threatened or involved by the infectious process.

Diagnosis	**Tissue**	**No. of lesions**	**Color**	**Size**	**Location**
Toxoplasmosis (**Figure 11**)	chorio-retina	1–3	White cream—new; usually near black—old scar, vitritis		Posterior pole, peripapillary
Toxocara (**Figure 12**)	Retina	One	White—elevated, TRD	1–2DD	Posterior pole
Tuberculosis	Choroid	1-multiple	Tuberculoma—white, round, elevated, indistinct margins, macular star	0.3–2DD	Posterior pole, midperiphery
Cytomegalovirus (CMV) (w or w/o HIV) (**Figure 13**)	Chorio-retina	Several	White areas with intraretinal hemorrhages, granular borders (Pizza pie)	Several DD	Everywhere
Acute retinal necrosis (herpetic) (**Figure 14**)	Retina	One	Confluent white-yellow, sharp irregular scalloped posterior margins, w or w/o intraretinal hemorrhages later replaced by atrophy and pigmentation	Several DD	Periphery
Syphilis	Sub-retina (chorio-retina)	Multiple, bilateral	Yellowish pale placoid lesions, optic nerve involvement	Variable	Anywhere, a mimicking disease
Cat scratch	Optic disc and retina		Optic disc edema with macular star	1–2 DD	Posterior pole
Candidiasis	Chorio-retina	Multiple	White faint with faint borders	0.5 DD	Posterior pole
Histoplasmosis	Choroid	Multiple	Small round lesions	0.2 DD	Anywhere

Table 1. TRD—traction retinal detachment; DD—disc diameter.

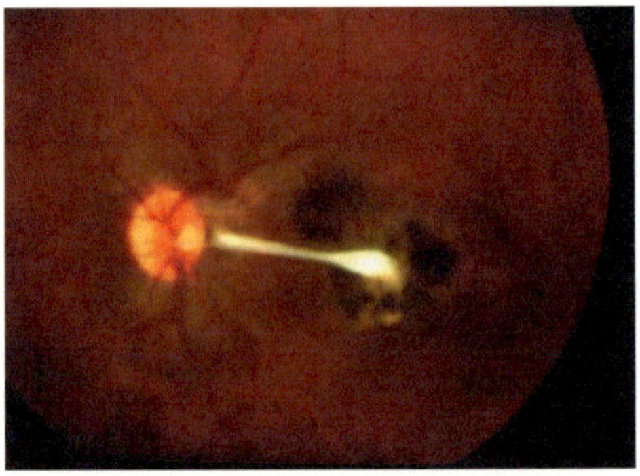

Figure 12. Toxocara chorioretinitis. Note the whitish lesion that may represent shrinked larva. Traction retinal detachment may occur.

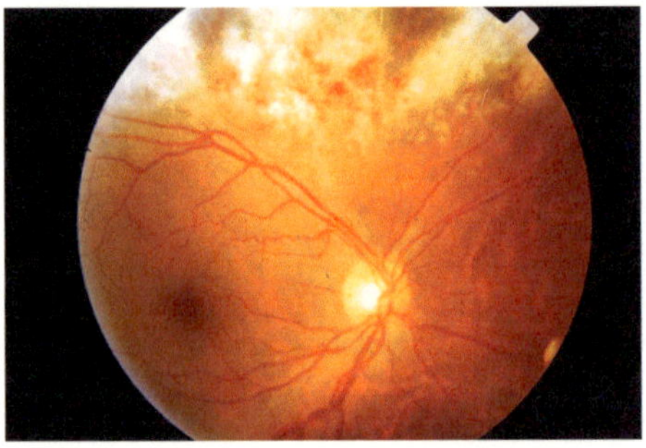

Figure 13. Cytomegalovirus (CMV) retinitis. Note the white lesions and intraretinal hemorrhages.

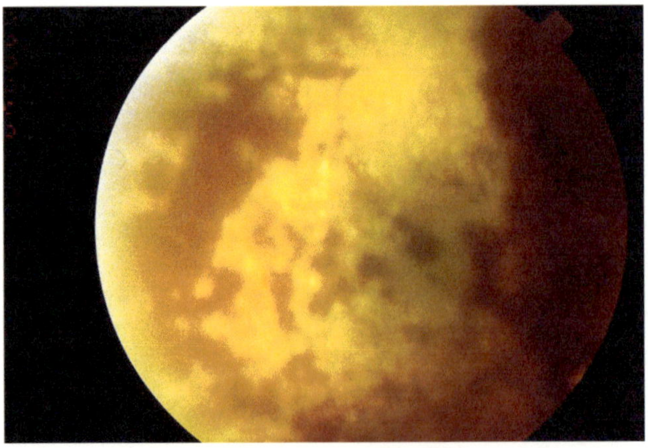

Figure 14. Acute retinal necrosis. Note the whitish lesion without retinal hemorrhages. The lesion is blurred by the inflammation in the vitreous.

7. Orbital infections

The hallmarks of orbital cellulitis include proptosis (exophthalmos) and limited ocular motility and/or involvement of the optic disc (decreased best-corrected visual acuity, positive afferent pupillary defect (Marcus Gunn) and/or swelling of the optic disc) [14, 15] (**Figure 15**). These findings differ from the signs of preseptal cellulitis in which swelling, erythema, heat and sensitivity of the eyelids occur. In both cases, the disease is usually unilateral. Orbital cellulitis in diabetic or immunocompromised patients should be considered as mucormycosis unless otherwise proven. Eschar of the oropharynx or the nose appears late and only in 10% of the patients with mucormycosis. Therefore, it should not be a sign to relay on. Bilateral orbital cellulitis may suggest of cavernous sinus thrombosis and diagnosis is made by computerized tomography. The clinical findings of cavernous sinus thrombosis are exophthalmos, unilateral or bilateral external and internal ophthalmoplegia that are usually accompanied by malaise and systemic fever (**Figure 16**). Nuchal rigidity as part of meningeal signs may also occur. Confirmation of the diagnosis is made by lumbar puncture. In orbital cellulitis and cavernous sinus thrombosis, blood cultures should be obtained when the body temperature increases to or over 39°C. In older patients, blood cultures are being obtained even if the temperature is normal. The source of the infection should be established by physical examination of the nose and mouth and imaging techniques (computed tomography and/or magnetic resonance imaging of the orbits and head. In contrast to preseptal cellulitis that is caused by infection from superficial skin wound, orbital cellulitis is most commonly caused by sinusitis (ethmoidal). Other sources may be upper jaw tooth abscess, otitis, mastoiditis, orbital osteomyelitis or extension from neglected preseptal cellulitis. Contamination may be by direct spreading through natural dehiscence sites and openings (foramina), veins, which are valveless or even nerves.

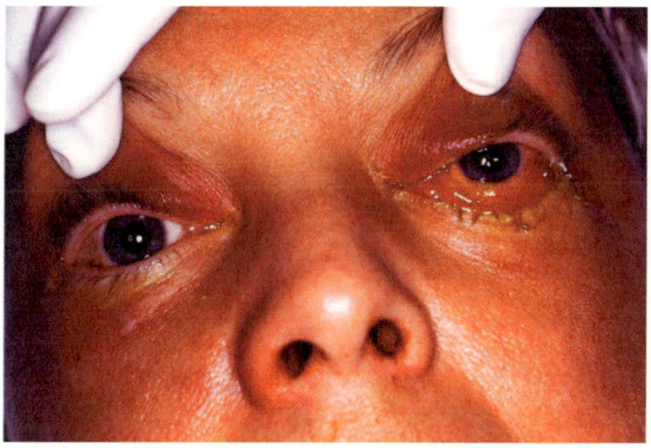

Figure 15. Cavernous sinus thrombosis in a diabetic patient. There was external ophthalmoplegia. The cause was mucormycosis.

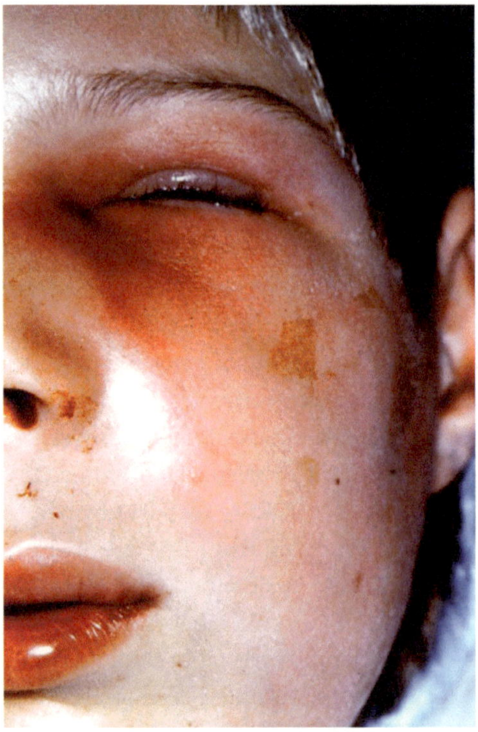

Figure 16. Orbital abscess as a result of tooth abscess. Note the erythema and swelling of both eyelids and chick.

Orbital abscess is a complication of orbital cellulitis (**Figure 16**) [16, 17]. It should be suspected when orbital cellulitis aggravates despite treatment. When aggravation occurs, repeated orbital computerized tomography assists in confirming the diagnosis of orbital abscess. In such a case, drainage of the abscess and continuing systemic antibiotics is required. The source of the infection should also be treated by surgical drainage. In cases of sinusitis, functional endoscopic sinus surgery (FESS) or other procedures with removal of the sinus mucosa may be required to prevent recurrences.

Note: The antibiotic dosage is for adults. The author is not responsible for the dosage or for any use of antibiotics.

Author details

Shimon Rumelt

Address all correspondence to: shimon.rumelt@naharia.health.gov.il

1 Western Galilee, Nahariya Medical Center, Nahariya, Israel

2 Faculty of Medicine, Bar Ilan University, Zefat, Israel

http://dx.doi.org/10.5772/65957

References

[1] Lederman C, Miller M. Hordeola and chalazia. Pediatr Rev 1999;20(8):283–284.

[2] Babar TF, Zaman M, Khan MN, Khan MD. Risk factors of preseptal and orbital cellulitis. J Coll Physicians Surg Pak 2009;19:39–42.

[3] Jackson WB. Blepharitis: current strategies for diagnosis and management. Can J Ophthalmol 2008;43:170–179.

[4] Hakkarainen TW, Kopari NM, Pham TN, Evans HL. Necrotizing soft tissue infections: review and current concepts in treatment, systems of care, and outcomes. Curr Probl Surg 2014;51:344–362.

[5] Raskin EM, Speaker MG, Laibson PR. Blepharitis. Infect Dis Clin North Am 1992;6:777–787.

[6] The Wills eye manual, 6th ed. 2012.

[7] Arfa RC, Grayson's diseases of the cornea, 3rd ed. St. Louis: Mosby. 1991.

[8] Guideline: American Academy of Ophthalmology cornea/external disease panel. Preferred Practice Pattern Guidelines. Conjunctivitis. San Francisco, CA. 2008.

[9] Panadero-Fontán R, Otranto D. Arthropods affecting the human eye. Vet Parasitol 2015; 208: 84–93.

[10] Park J, Lee KM, Zhou H, Rabin M, Jwo K, Burton WB, et al. Community practice patterns for bacterial corneal ulcer evaluation and treatment. Eye Contact Lens 2015;41:12–18.

[11] Rowsey JJ, Jensen H, Sexton DJ. Clinical diagnosis of endophthalmitis. Int Ophthalmol Clin 1987;27:82–88.

[12] Sudharshan S, Ganesh SK, Biswas J. Current approach in the diagnosis and management of posterior uveitis. Indian J Ophthalmol 2010;58:29–43.

[13] Khairallah M, Chee SP, Rathinam SR, Attia S, Nadella V. Novel infectious agents causing uveitis. Int Ophthalmol 2010;30:465–483.

[14] Bergin DJ, Wright JE. Orbital cellulitis. Br J Ophthalmol 1986;70:174–178.

[15] Rumelt S, Rubin PA. Potential sources of orbital cellulitis. Int Ophthalmol Clin 1996;36:207–221.

[16] Harris GJ. Subperiosteal abscess of the orbit. Arch Ophthalmol 1983;101:751–757.

[17] Liao JC, Harris GJ. Subperiosteal abscess of the orbit: evolving pathogens and the therapeutic protocol. Ophthalmology 2015;122:639–647.

Section 2

Specific Clinical Intities

Chapter 2

Bacterial Endophthalmitis

S. Malhotra, S. Sharma, N. J. K. Bhatia, C. Hans and P. Kumar

Additional information is available at the end of the chapter

http://dx.doi.org/10.5772/61608

Abstract

Endophthalmitis is an ocular inflammation involving vitreous cavity along with the retinal and uveal components of the eye mostly due to infectious agent. The source of infection could be exogenous or endogenous. Exogenous endophthalmitis results from direct inoculation as a complication of ocular surgery, foreign bodies or penetrating ocular trauma, while endogenous endophthalmitis results from haematogenous spread of organisms from a distant source of infection. Endophthalmitis often results in partial or complete loss of vision despite aggressive therapeutic and surgical intervention and hence it is considered as a medical emergency. Diagnosis of infectious agent is critical in the management of these agents. Intravitreal antimicrobial therapy along with anti-inflammatory agents is the key ingredient for successful management of endophthalmitis, while surgical procedures like vitrectomy become necessary in severe endophthalmitis cases. This is a brief review regarding classification, etiological agents causing endophthalmitis, diagnosis and therapeutic challenges of endophthalmitis that will help in improving the visual outcome.

Keywords: Bacterial endophthalmitis, diagnosis, therapeutic challenge

1. Introduction

Endophthalmitis is an ocular inflammation into the posterior segment of the eye usually involving vitreous cavity along with the retinal and uveal components of the eye [1] due to infectious agent, usually bacterial or fungal or non-infectious causes. Normally, the blood–ocular barrier prevents invasion from infective organisms, but if this is breached (directly through trauma or indirectly due to a change in its permeability secondary to inflammation), infection can occur. Endophthalmitis often results in partial or complete loss of vision despite aggressive therapeutic and surgical intervention and hence it is considered as a medical emergency [2, 3]. When inflammation spreads throughout the globe involving all the layers including the Tenon's capsule with or without involvement of the peri-ocular tissues, the condition is known as panophthalmitis. Hence, in endophthalmitis there is involvement of all ocular tissues except the sclera while in panophthalmitis there is involvement of all ocular tissues including the sclera. Panophthalmitis is a devastating fulminant condition associated with complete loss of vision and with very poor prognosis [3].

Features	Infectious endophthalmitis	Non-infectious endophthalmitis
Symptoms	Severe vision loss with moderate to severe pain.	Vision loss is mild to moderate with mild pain.
Signs	Conjunctival congestion is seen along with hypopyon and fibrin deposits. Also vitreous opacity is prominent.	Conjunctival congestion, hypopyon and fibrin deposits are usually not seen. Vitreous opacity is usually mild.
Slit lamp examination	Retinal infiltrates and intra-retinal haemorrhages are common.	Retinal infiltrates and intra-retinal haemorrhages are very rarely seen.
Clinical course	Rapidly progressive.	Slow improvement.
Treatment	Antibiotics and surgery.	Topical and/or systemic corticosteroids.

Table 1. Difference between infectious and non-infectious endophthalmitis [4]

2. Sterile/non-infectious endophthalmitis

Sterile endophthalmitis is an acute intra-ocular inflammation of the vitreous cavity that resolves without the need of intra-vitreal antibiotics and/or vitreo-retinal surgery. In these cases if vitreous microbiological study is done, it needs to be culture negative. This condition has diverse etiologies and includes systemic auto-immune diseases, local ocular inflammations of unknown cause, endophthalmitis related to lens material and endophthalmitis attributable to intra-ocular foreign bodies.

Phacoanaphylactic endophthalmitis (lens-induced granulomatous inflammation) is a type of non-infectious endophthalmitis which represents an auto-immune response to lens protein. This is a rare consequence of lens injury which may occur after trauma causing rupturing of the lens capsule, or post surgery such as following extracapsular cataract extraction when residual lens cortex is present. There is a mixed neutrophilic and granulomatous response seen around the lens in histology [5].

Phacotoxic endophthalmitis is a condition which was previously used to cover a mixed group of conditions related to cataract surgery and intra-ocular lens implant surgery. However, since inflammation is seen mostly in the anterior segment, the term was changed to toxic anterior segment syndrome (TASS). TASS is caused due to reactions to chemicals (irrigationsolutions, preservatives, drugs, denatured viscoelastics), IOL (intra-ocular lens) materials, instrument sterilization and preparation-related compounds [6,7]. TASS presents with marked decrease in vision and diffuse corneal oedema within 12–24 h of anterior segment surgery, most commonly cataract surgery and, more recently, it has been reported after phakic intra-ocular lens implantation [6,8].

Sterile endophthalmitis has also been noted following intra-ocular injection, post vitrectomy and after glaucoma drainage device implantation surgery. Intra-vitreal triamcinolone acetonide has also been associated with sterile endophthalmitis when triamcinolone crystals migrate into the anterior chamber [9]. Clinically, sterile endophthalmitis presents within 24 h of surgery, Gram stain and culture negative, involving the anterior segment in the case of TASS, and showing no response to antibiotics but improvement is seen with topical and/or oral steroids. However, it is difficult to rule out infectious etiology because some infectious cases mayhave rapid onset and have initial negative cultures [6].

3. Classification of bacterial endopthalmitis

Endophthalmitis can be categorized as exogenous and endogenous endophthalmitis. Exogenous endophthalmitis results from direct inoculation as a complication of any intra-ocular surgery (**post-operative endophthalmitis**) and/or blunt or penetrating ocular trauma (**post-traumatic endophthalmitis**). Destruction of intra-ocular tissues may be due to direct invasion by the organism and/or inflammatory mediators of the immune response. **Endogenous endophthalmitis** results from the haematogenous spread of organisms from a distant source of infection [10]. Rarely, keratitis (infection of the cornea), if left untreated, can result in corneal perforation and intra-ocular seeding of organisms leading to endophthalmitis [11]. According to British report, 59% of endophthalmitis were exogenous while 41% were endogenous in origin [12]. In comparison, another study from India suggested that 92.6% were exogenous endophthalmitis and only 7.4% were endogenous endophthalmitis [13]. There are multiple factors responsible for variation in incidence, namely, number of patients included in the study, duration of study, urban versus rural population, pre-disposing factors present, inpatient versus outpatient population and geographical areas of study.

3.1. Post-operative endophthalmitis

Post-operative endophthalmitis is the most common form of endopthalmitis and it occurs most frequently following cataract surgeries like phacoemulsification and intra-ocular lens implantation. However, other procedures namely corneal surgeries (penetrating keratoplasty, keratoprosthesis insertion, refractive corneal surgeries), vitreous procedures (intra-vitreal injections, vitrectomies), glaucoma surgical treatments (blebs, glaucoma valve placements), procedures to correct retinal detachment including scleral buckling, and strabismus correction are also associated with varying risks of endophthalmitis. The organisms are generally acquired from eyelid margin and pre-ocular tear film [2,3]. Contributing factors for development of endophthalmitis include dry eye, corneal perforation, systemic immune dysfunction, previous presence of infection like bacterial conjunctivitis, cicatricial disorders (e.g. ocular cicatricial pemphigoid and Steven-Johnson), chronic use of topical antibiotics and both topical and oral corticosteroid use [11]. In various vitrectomies (Pars plana vitrectomy or 25 gauge vitrectomy), diabetes mellitus is recognized as an important risk factor for exogenous endophthalmitis [14]. Sometimes, cases of clustering of the endophthalmitis are seen, suggesting contaminated materials/solutions or problems with instrument sterilization as responsible [15,

16]. Bacterial infections are the most common cause of post-operative endophthalmitis, and Gram-positive isolates account for the majority of these cases [2]. Coagulase negative *Staphylococcus* accounts for majority of cases followed by *enterococci* and *streptococci* of viridans group. Among Gram-negative isolates, *Pseudomonas aeruginosa* endophthalmitis is identified [17, 18]. Fungal infections are less common and occur particularly in association with the use of contaminated ocular irrigation fluids [19]. *Candida* spp. (especially *C. parapsilosis*), *Aspergillus* spp. and *Fusarium* spp. are common fungal pathogens responsible for post-operative endophthalmitis [20]. *E. faecalis* is the causative agent in 4% to 8% of post-operative endophthalmitis cases and is isolated most frequently from infected filtering blebs following glaucoma surgery [10]. The visual outcome is poor and has become a key public health concern because of the emergence of antibiotic resistance to useful antibiotics including vancomycin [21].

Delayed onset infection (> 6 weeks post-operative) may occur due to sequesteration of low-virulence organisms introduced at the time of surgery or to delayed inoculation of organisms [22, 23]. *S. epidermidis, Propionibacterium acnes,* filamentous bacteria (including *Actinomyces* and *Nocardia* sp.), *Hemophilus influenzae,* non-tuberculous mycobacteria (*M. abscessus, M. chelonae* etc.) and *candida* spp. are responsible for chronic or delayed endophthalmitis [24, 25]. In cases with delayed onset infection, organisms gain access to the eye through either wound abnormalities, suture tracks or filtering blebs. It is more common with glaucoma filtering surgery [26].

3.2. Post-traumatic endophthalmitis

Penetrating injuries are accompanied by higher infection rate of 1–17% compared to post-surgery cases [10]. The broad prevalence range is due to factors such as frequency of intra-ocular foreign bodies, distribution of trauma causes, and management strategies. Onset may be acute or delayed, but the most virulent organisms can destroy an eye within hours. Important risk factors for post-traumatic endophthalmitis are the presence of an intra-ocular foreign body (IOFB), the length of time between injury and foreign body removal, delay in closure of the globe, poorer visual acuity at presentation, virulence of organisms and the immune system of the affected individual [27]. Post-traumatic-endophthalmitis-associated isolates are mostly derived from the environment, and hence includes greater variety of organisms than those following ocular surgery. *Staphylococcus* and *Streptococcus* sp. are the most frequent pathogens, followed by *Bacillus cereus and P. aeruginosa* [28]. Filamentous fungi, especially *Aspergillus* sp. and *Fusarium* sp., are also responsible for post-traumatic endophthalmitis [29]. Bacillus infection is noteworthy as it causes rapid destruction of eye leading to decline in retinal function and vision loss within 24 to 48 h post-infection, despite aggressive treatment and/or surgical intervention. This suggests that even if the infected eye is rendered sterile by antibiotics, ocular damage continues to occur due to the bacterial toxins produced – haemolysins, lipases, enterotoxins and proteases – acting together [30].

3.3. Endogenous endophthalmitis

Endogenous endophthalmitis is relatively rare accounting for 2% to 8% of all endophthalmitis cases [31]. It results from the introduction of organisms into the eye as a result of haematoge-

http://dx.doi.org/10.5772/61608

nous spread from a remote primary site of infection [31]. Populations at greatest risk include immunocompromised patients like diabetes, HIV, organ transplant, cardiac disease and malignancy or those on immunosuppressive therapy, patients with prolonged indwelling devices and intra-venous drug abusers [32]. Endogenous endophthalmitis is more common with fungal isolates than with bacterial isolates. Most common fungal pathogens include *Candida* spp., *Aspergillus* sp. and *Fusarium* spp. *Candida albicans* remains the most important although others such as *C. glabrata, C. tropicalis, C. dubliniensis* and *C. krusei* are being increasingly detected [33]. *Aspergillus* sp. (*A. fumigatus* followed by *A. flavus*) have been reported less frequently than *Candida* sp., but Aspergillus endophthalmitis cause rapidly progressive retinal damage and is more visually devastating compared to Candida endophthalmitis [34]. Common causes of endogenous bacterial endophthalmitis include *S. aureus, B. cereus* and Gram-negative organisms, including *Escherichia coli, Neisseria meningitidis* and *Klebsiella* spp. [10]. *Bacillus* spp. is a primary cause of endogenous endophthalmitis in intra-venous drug abusers due to contaminated injections and drug solutions [10]. Rarely, protozoa like Microsporidia and Amoebae may be the pathogens for endogenous endophthalmitis [35]. It is seen that visual outcomes are poorer with endogenous fungal endophthalmitis compared to endogenous bacterial endophthalmitis. The common foci of infection may be urinary tract infection, septic arthritis, pneumonia and endocarditis [35]. Seriously ill patients may neglect eye symptoms until vision is permanently compromised. Hence, it has been recommended that ophthalmic screening should be routine in high-risk situations such as intra-venous drug use, long-term antibiotics, immunosuppressive therapy, primary or secondary immunodeficiency, prolonged central line use, debilitated patients and pre-mature infants [36].

3.3.1. Endophthalmitis associated with microbial keratitis

Cornea gets infected in situations like contact lens wearer, any pre-existing corneal disease and rarely due to dry cornea (as seen in chronic blepharoconjunctivitis or dacrocystitis, tear film deficiency or topical steroid therapy). If corneal infection is severe enough to cause progressive ulceration of cornea, then it can lead to bacterial endophthalmitis [11].

The incidence rates [37, 38] and etiologial agents of different types of endophthalmitis have been enumerated in Tables 2 and 3, respectively.

Source of infection	**Causes**	**Incidence rate**
Exogenous endophthalmitis		
1. Post-operative	Overall	0.05–0.3%
	Post-cataract surgery	0.02–0.11%
	Post-intravitreal injection	0.03–0.87%
	Post-penetrating keratoplasty	0.1–0.5%
	Post-keratoprostheses	0–12.5%
	Glaucoma valve surgery	1.7–1.9%
	Filtering blebs	0.2–9.6%

Source of infection	Causes	Incidence rate
	Vitrectomy	0.05–0.14%
	Episcleral surgery	0.01%
	Strabismus surgery	Very rare (1 in 30,000)
1. Post-traumatic		1–17%
Endogenous endophthalmitis		2–8%

Table 2. Incidence rates of different types of endophthalmitis

Source of infection	**Classification**	Causative agents
Exogenous	**1. Post-operative endophthalmitis**	
	Acute (within 6 weeks of surgery)	Coagulase-negative staphylococci (Most common "/>60%), *Staphylococcus aureus*, viridans group streptococci, and enterococci. Gram-negative organisms like *Pseudomonas aeruginosa* [2]. Fungi like *Candida* spp. (especially *C. parapsilosis*), *Aspergillus* spp. and *Fusarium* spp.
	Delayed or chronic (after 6 weeks of surgery)	*Propionibacterium acne* (most common), *Streptococcus* spp., coagulase negative staphylococci (*S. epidermidis*), filamentous bacteria (including *Actinomyces and Nocardia* sp.), *Hemophilus influenzae*, non-tuberculous mycobacteria (*M. abscessus, M. chelonae*, etc.) and *candida* spp. (*Candida parapsilosis*).
	2. Post-traumatic endophthalmitis	Staphylococci (most common), *Bacillus cereus, Streptococci, P. aeruginosa* and polymicrobial infections. Filamentous fungi, especially *Aspergillus* sp. and *Fusarium* sp.
Endogenous	**Endogenous endophthalmitis**	Fungi like *Candida spp. (Candida albicans, C. glabrata, C. tropicalis, C. dubliniensis, C. krusei), Aspergillus* sp. (*A. fumigatus, A. flavus*) and *Fusarium* spp. Gram-positive bacteria include *S. aureus, B. cereus* and Gram-negative organisms, including *Escherichia coli, Neisseria meningitidis* and *Klebsiella* spp. Rarely, protozoa like Microsporidia and Amoebae.

Table 3. Etiological agents of different types of endophthalmitis

4. Clinical presentation

Clinical presentation of the disease depends on the virulence and toxin production of the infecting pathogen, the mechanism of introduction into the eye, how quickly treatment is initiated and the patient's age [10]. Symptoms of endophthalmitis range from a relatively painless anterior chamber inflammation, such as that typically caused by *Staphylococcus epidermidis* to an indolent and protracted intra-ocular infection caused by *P. acnes,* to an explosive ocular and periorbital infection caused by *B. cereus* [10]. The clinical presentations of various endophthalmitis are depicted in Table 4.

Types	Symptoms	Signs
Acute post-operative endophthalmitis	• Sudden decrease of vision and increasing eye pain • Red eye, ocular discharge and blurring of vision [38, 39].	• Lid oedema, intense conjunctival injection and chemosis, corneal oedema, papillary fibrin membrane and hypopyon [Figures 1 and 2]. • Severe inflammation in the anterior chamber and the vitreous [38, 39].
Delayed post-operative endophthalmitis	• Insidious decrease of vision and gradually increasing redness with minimal pain [40].	• Conjunctival injection, hypopyon, corneal oedema and clumps of exudates on the iris or around the pupillary margin.
Bleb associated endophthalmitis	• Rapidly worsening pain and vision • Red eye	• Marked conjunctival injection and hypopyon. • Bleb appears milky white with area of necrosis in the sclera (Figure 3).
Post-traumatic endophthalmitis	Same as acute post-operative endophthalmitis, but more severe and early onset in *Bacillus cereus* infection (Figure 4).	Same as acute post-operative endophthalmitis • Fever, proptosis and corneal oedema [38, 39].
Endogenous endophthalmitis	• Acutely ill immunocompromised patient presenting with decreased vision	• Lid and conjunctival oedema • Flame-shaped retinal haemorrhages. • Hypopyon, vitreous inflammatory reaction and microabscesses on the iris [39].
Candida endogenous endophthalmitis	• Decreased vision, floaters and pain • Usually bilateral and follow an indolent course	• Fluffy yellow white retinal lesions and retinal haemorrhages. • Hypopyon and widespread inflammation.

Table 4. Clinical presentation of various endophthalmitis

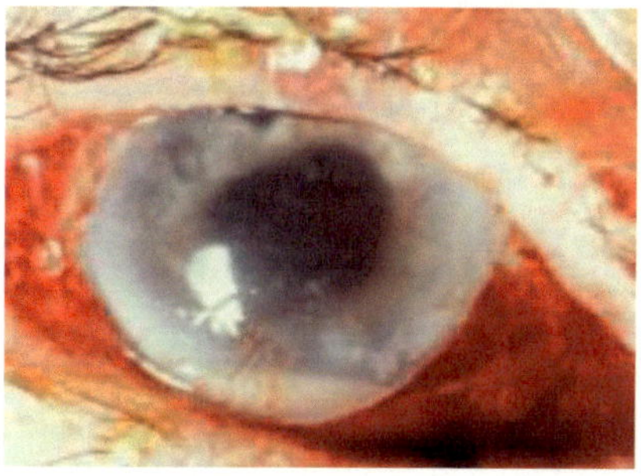

Figure 1. Intense conjunctival congestion with corneal edema and hypopyon

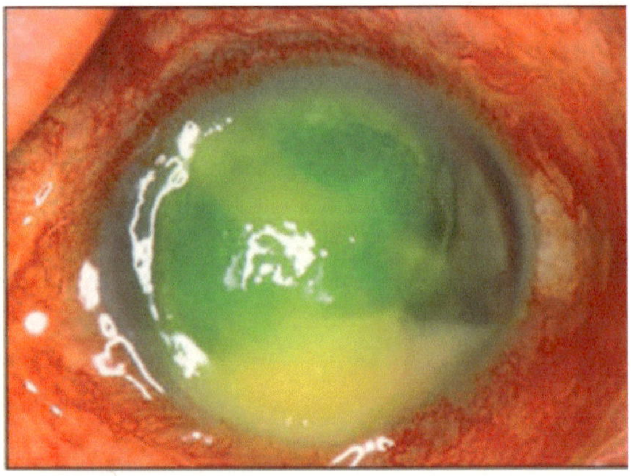

Figure 2. Endophthalmitis affecting the cornea

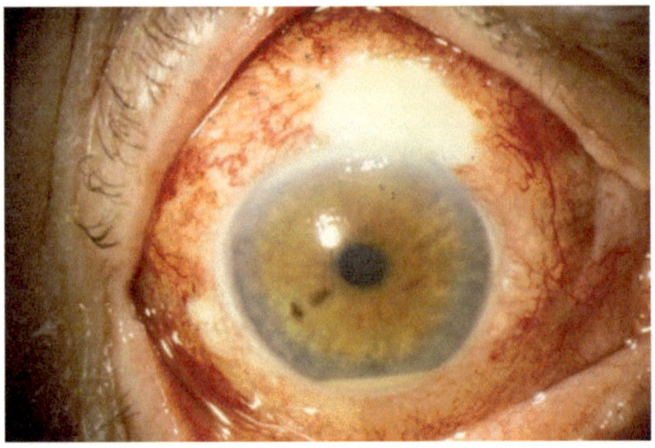

Figure 3. White bleb with intense conjunctival injection suggestive of bleb-associated endophthalmitis

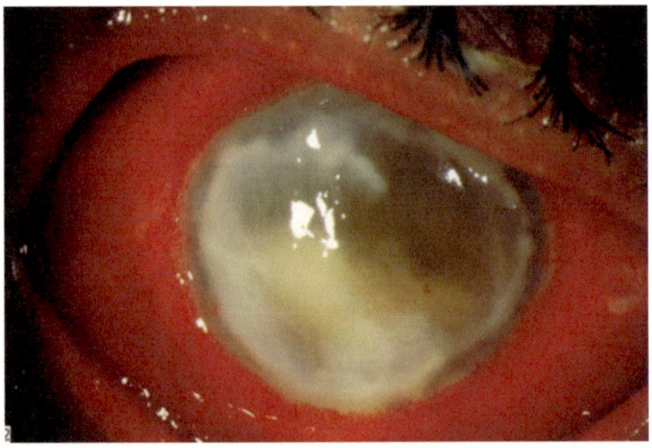

Figure 4. Post-traumatic endophthalmitis caused by *Bacillus cereus* showing prominent conjunctival congestion, corneal ring infiltrate and dense hypopyon

http://dx.doi.org/10.5772/61608

5. Pathogenesis of bacterial endophthalmitis

5.1. Protective mechanisms in eye

5.1.1. Blood–ocular fluid barrier

Under normal circumstances, the blood–ocular barrier provides a natural resistance against invading organisms and it ensures proper functioning of intra-ocular tissues and is essential for immune privilege [10]. The blood–ocular fluid barrier consists of inner and outer blood–retina barriers and the blood–aqueous humour barrier. The inner blood–retina barrier is formed by tight junctions between the endothelial cells and basement membrane of retinal capillaries and retinal pericytes, which control the blood supply for the inner retinal layers, preventing leakage of plasma constituents into the vitreous. The tight junctions between retinal pigment epithelial cells constitute the outer blood–retina barrier and control the blood supply to retinal photoreceptor cells and the choriocapillaris. The blood aqueous humour barrier is formed by the iris and ciliary epithelium and thus divides the highly perfused iris from its neighbouring compartments, the anterior chamber and the anterior vitreous [41]. Certain cytokines, such as transforming growth factor β, α-melanocyte stimulating hormone and vasoactive intestinal peptide, are known to have immunosuppressive property and have been detected in healthy aqueous humour [10].

5.1.2. Anterior Chamber-Associated Immune Deviation (ACAID)

Ocular antigen presenting cells, namely macrophages and dendritic cells, are found in the iris and the choriocapillaris [42]. In most cases of post-operative endophthalmitis, bacteria enter the eye via the anterior chamber, where antigen presentation initially occurs and hence antigen presenting cells residing in the iris are the most likely to first encounter these pathogens. This process may be facilitated by the mild inflammatory reaction in the anterior segment, resulting from tissue manipulation of surgery. Retinal and uveal antigen presenting cells may not have access to antigen under physiological conditions but can activate during the later stages of infection, if the microbes have gained access to the posterior segment. When the defense mechanisms of immune privilege are overwhelmed, then only fulminant inflammation occurs [10].

5.1.3. Invading mechanisms of organisms

Organisms causing endophthalmitis are mostly part of conjunctival flora. They adhere to IOLs and create microcolonies through biofilm formation and within biofilms they are protected from host inflammatory responses, both physically and through multiple genetic changes that alter antigenicity. Organisms in the biofilm are thus difficult to eradicate and may persist despite antibiotic treatment, resulting in relapsing endophthalmitis [43].

Various toxins and enzymes are produced and secreted by the invading organisms causing destruction of protective mechanisms in the eye in case of fulminant infection in eye. *B. cereus* produces a number of cytolysins and enzymes that could contribute to the rapid course and severity of endophthalmitis, including haemolysins, lipases, enterotoxins and proteases

[30]. *E. faecalis* strains frequently harbour conjugative plasmids that encode a cytolysin which effectively lyses both eukaryotic and prokaryotic cells [44]. Cytolysin causes destructive changes in retinal architecture and vitreal structures. Adhesin, aggregation substance, produced by enterococci is a virulence-enhancing factor and helps them to attach to membranous vitreous structures. *S. aureus* secretes cell wall-associated products and adhesions (e.g. clumping factor, fibronectin-binding protein and protein A) and extracellular virulence factors (e.g. toxins such as alpha-toxin, beta-toxin, gamma-toxin and leukocidin, proteases and lipases) which are responsible for high virulence of this organism in endophthalmitis. These virulence factors are controlled by quorum-sensing systems namely, *agr* (accessory gene regulator) and *sar* (staphylococcal accessory regulator) [45]. Hence, therapeutics designed to inactivate global regulation of *S. aureus* during the early stages of infection may be more effective in arresting tissue damage than targeting individual toxins.

6. Role of complement and proinflammatory cytokines in endophthalmitis

IL-1 initially mediates the acute-phase response, inducing other inflammatory mediators such as prostaglandins, phospholipase A2, collagenases and other proinflammatory cytokines (IL-6 and tumour necrosis factor alpha [TNF-α]). IL-1 induces the breakdown of the blood–retina barrier and leukocyte recruitment into the intra-ocular tissue [10]. IL-6 induces production of acute phase proteins such as C-reactive protein and fibrinogen by the liver and promotes B- and T-cell differentiation [46]. In the eye, IL-6 plays a local role in negative feedback on IL-1 and TNF-α production. TNF-α also provokes an intra-ocular inflammatory reaction and acts synergistically with IL-1. IL-8 promotes the recruitment of neutrophils, and because dense neutrophil infiltration is a characteristic feature of endophthalmitis, its involvement in intra-ocular infection is probable but has not yet been determined [10].

7. Brief overview of pathogenesis

During bacterial growth, toxin production by virulent organisms results in loss of retinal function. Cell envelopes, fragments of peptidoglycan, and teichoic acid or lipopolysaccharides are released in intra-ocular spaces during intra-ocular growth or antibiotic killing. These components may come in contact with resident immune cells and stimulate them to produce pro-inflammatory cytokines or other immune mediators which initiate a cascade of inflammatory events, including increased permeability of the blood–ocular fluid barrier, with influx of additional soluble mediators and recruitment of phagocytic inflammatory cells to the site of infection. Inflammatory cells may in turn produce more inflammatory cytokines, in addition to toxic enzymes and reactive oxygen species. During the later stages of protracted endophthalmitis, lymphocytes migrate into inflamed intra-ocular tissues, and an immunoglobulin response results as shown in Figure 5. The ultimate result is the disruption of retinal architecture and death of non-regenerating retinal photoreceptor cells and a significant intra-ocular inflammatory response which can exacerbate the harmful effects of bacterial growth and toxin production by causing bystander damage [10].

http://dx.doi.org/10.5772/61608

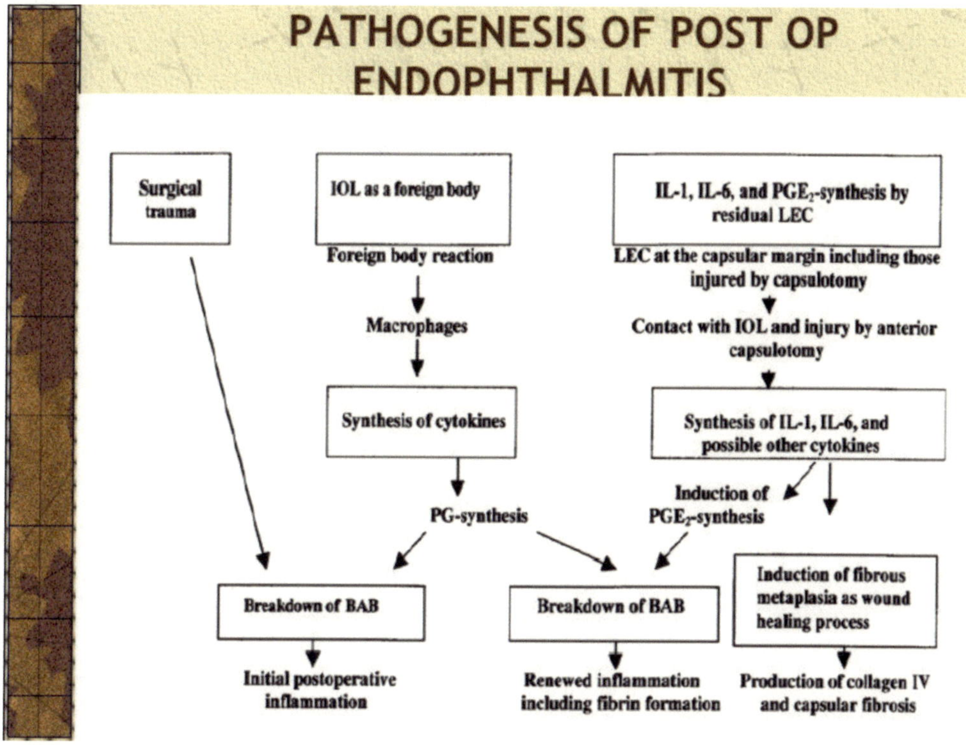

Figure 5. Brief overview of pathogenesis of bacterial endophthalmitis

7.1. Diagnosis of bacterial endophthalmitis

7.1.1. Laboratory diagnosis

The clinical diagnosis of endophthalmitis is confirmed by obtaining intra-ocular specimens like aqueous and vitreous specimen [47]. The possibility of isolating a microorganism from the vitreous specimen is 56–70%, whereas it is 36–40% from the anterior chamber (AC) humour [48]. Culture and sensitivity studies on aqueous and vitreous samples are necessary to determine the type of organism and antibiotic sensitivity.[9, 10] If endogenous bacterial endophthalmitis is suspected, a systemic workup for the source of infection is required, with cultures of blood, sputum and urine. Anterior chamber tap can be done by introducing 30-gauge needle on a tuberculin syringe to anterior chamber through limbus to obtain a 0.1 ml sample under topical anesthesia. The vitreous specimen can be obtained either by vitreous tap, vitreous biopsy or by using an automated vitrectomy instrument. In vitreous tap, a 21-gauge needle on a tuberculin syringe is used to obtain 0.1–0.2 ml of vitreous sample under sub-Tenon block. Vitreous biopsy can be taken using a 23-gauge vitrectomy cutter. Direct inoculation of the intra-ocular fluid specimen onto specific culture media is especially important when limited specimens are obtained. Specimens obtained with automated vitrectomy instruments can be processed by two methods. Vitrectomy specimen is either passed through 0.45 mm filter paper that concentrates the microorganisms and particulate matter and filter paper is sectioned and distributed on the appropriate media or vitrectomy specimen is directly inoculated into standard blood culture bottle [49]. Specimens can be inoculated on 5% sheep blood agar for recovery of the most common bacterial and fungal isolates. Sabouraud dextrose agar is also inoculated for recovery of fungal isolates. Chocolate agar: can be used for the recovery of fastidious organisms (i.e. *Neisseria gonorrhoeae* and *Hemophilus influenzae*). Thioglycollate broth and anaerobic blood agar are useful for recovery of small numbers of aerobic or anaerobic (including *Propionibacterium acnes*) organisms from ocular fluids and tissues. Blood culture bottles contain specially prepared medium for the recovery of both aerobic and anaerobic bacteria and fungi and it can be directly inoculated by intra-ocular fluids. Immunologic and molecular genetic technologies enable rapid and specific identification of infectious agents. In culture negative cases, the additional use of polymerase chain reaction was reported to aid in the identification of the organism [49]. These real-time techniques have been used in both clinical and experimental settings, and their future use in this area appears promising [50, 51].

In the Endophthalmitis Vitrectomy Study (EVS), Gram stain result did not reveal any subgroups in which vitrectomy had a beneficial value and therefore is not useful in making initial therapeutic decisions [26]. Also in EVS, there was no difference in the culture positivity rate and operative complications between samples obtained by tap and those obtained by vitrectomy [52].

7.1.2. Imaging studies

In B-scan ultrasound of the posterior pole, choroidal thickening and ultrasound echoes in the vitreous support the diagnosis of endophthalmitis. Retained lens material and associated retinal detachment are also visible. The ultrasound also provides a baseline prior to intra-ocular intervention and allows assessment of the posterior vitreous face and areas of possible traction [53]. In traumatic cases, a CT scan can be performed, which may show thickening of the sclera and uveal tissues associated with various degrees of increased density in the vitreous and peri-ocular soft tissue structures. In endogenous cases, imaging modalities like two-dimensional echocardiography and chest x-ray can be done to rule out potential sources of infection.

8. Prevention of endophthalmitis

The most effective therapy for endophthalmitis is prevention. Sterile technique during any type of ocular surgery is important. All instruments for surgery should be thoroughly sterilized with autoclaving; tubing is preferably sterilized with ethylene oxide gas sterilizer. BSS (balanced salt solution) bottles should never be kept or used for more than one operating session. Proper preparation before any intra-ocular surgery including peri-ocular and ocular surface (cul-de-sac) sterilization with povidone iodine 5% applied for 3 min is the best means for prevention of endophthalmitis (superior to topical antibiotics) [54]. In allergic patients, 0.05% chlorhexidine can be used. Large bottles of diluted povidone iodine or chlorhexidine should be avoided and single-use vials be used as they get contaminated with *P. aeruginosa*. A prophylactic antibiotic like topical 0.5% levofloxacin or ofloxacin one drop 1 h and one drop 30 min before surgery and three drops at 5 min intervals immediately following surgery is effective in reducing the rate of post-operative endophthalmitis according to the European Society of Cataract and Refractive Surgery (ESCRS) study [55]. Topical antibiotic should be continued four times a day for two weeks post-operatively. The use of antibiotics in the irrigation and infusion fluid is also an option. In addition, washing the surgical gloves whether containing talc or not, after wearing them in sterile saline and washing any surgical instrument before introducing it into the eye and avoiding touching any non-sterile place including the body surface with anything. Biodegradable scleral plugs impregnated with antibiotics, antiviral and anti-inflammatory drugs have been tested for drug release *in vitro*. Scleral plugs containing vancomycin, amikacin and dexamethasone have been used for slow delivery of drugs in the vitreal cavity at a concentration well above MIC (minimum inhibitory concentration) for a period of time needed to treat bacterial endophthalmitis in place of repeated vitreal injections [56, 57]. All patients with ocular penetration injuries should be treated with IV broad-spectrum antibiotics for 3 days. The common regimen is cefazolin 1 g tds and gentamycin 80 mg BD. If injury is through contaminated object, vancomycin 1 g bd (in slow infusion to prevent "red man" syndrome) should substitute cefazolin. In patients allergic to penicillins or cephalosporins, moxifloxacin 400 mg once a day may be used.

8.1. Treatment strategy for endophthalmitis

Endophthalmitis is an ocular emergency, and urgent treatment is required to reduce the potential of significant visual loss. Microbial endophthalmitis is a therapeutic challenge due to delicate anatomy and physiology of ocular tissues. Retina has a rich blood supply, but the vitreous and anterior chambers are avascular and are isolated from systemic circulation via blood–ocular fluid barrier [4]. These features represent a barrier for the delivery of cellular and humoral mediators of host immunity and also antimicrobial or anti-inflammatory agents administered systemically. This leaves clinicians with few treatment options like injecting drug directly into intra-ocular space, but there is a risk of vitreous or sub-retinal haemorrhaging, retinal toxicity, corneal abrasions, central artery occlusion, uveitis or lens opacification [58]. Also, retinal photoreceptor cells are highly sensitive not only to the offending pathogen and the resulting inflammatory response but also to antimicrobial agents administered locally to treat the infection [59].

8.2. Antimicrobial agents and anti-inflammatory agents

Outcome of endophthalmitis management depends on several factors, including the responsible pathogen, the patient's age, the duration between injury and treatment, the therapy chosen and the condition of the eye upon presentation [60]. Delay in therapy results in poor visual outcome, especially in severe cases of endophthalmitis. Bacterial endophthalmitis is treated with repeated injection of antibiotics into the vitreous concurrently with systemic antibiotics, although some potentially effective antibiotics like vancomycin and aminoglycosides do not penetrate readily into the vitreous, due to the protective effect of the blood–ocular fluid barrier; however, intra-ocular inflammation increases the permeability of the blood–

ocular fluid barrier, enhancing penetration of systemic antibiotics into the vitreous cavity [61]. Another reason for poor systemic antibiotic effect in endophthalmitis is poor penetration through the blood flow because of the inflammation and necrosis of blood vessels. Because of variable penetration into the vitreous cavity of aminoglycosides, vancomycin and cephalosporins, the EVS evaluated their clinical efficacy in a post-cataract surgery endophthalmitis controlled trial and found that systemic antibiotics did not enhance visual outcomes in these patients. However, this recommendation does not hold true following other types of ocular surgery, trauma or suspected endogenous endophthalmitis [62]. Systemic antibiotics are important for therapeutic management of endogenous endophthalmitis where there is concomitant bacteremia, while intravitreal antibiotic is a key component for clinical management of exogenous bacterial endophthalmitis. Fluoroquinolones are currently used by many clinicians in combination with intravitreal antibiotics like vancomycin, amikacin and ceftazidime for severe endophthalmitis cases. The two drug regimens commonly used by clinicians include vancomycin (1 mg/0.1 ml) to cover Gram-positive organisms and a third-generation cephalosporin (ceftazidime 2 mg /0.1 ml) or amikacin (0.4 mg/0.1 ml) to cover Gram-negative organisms [63]. Repeated intravitreal injections of antibiotics may be necessary if there is no response to the initial therapy.

Fungal endophthalmitis carries a poor prognosis and there is no standard management available for treating this condition. In fungal endophthalmitis cases, systemic antifungal agents namely amphotericin with or without flucytosine or fluconazole are used. In fluconazole-resistant strains voriconazole may be helpful; however, information on new antifungal agents for endophthalmitis is limited. It is seen that chorioretinitis infections can be more readily cured with systemic antifungal agents, whereas more aggressive treatment including pars plana vitrectomy with intravitreal amphotericin (5–10mg/0.1mL) or voriconazole and systemic antifungal is required for patients with vitritis. Topical antifungal agents (natamycin 5%) are also included, especially in cases of corneal involvement [64].

The use of corticosteroids is controversial. In endophthalmitis, ocular inflammation is induced by growing bacteria and also due to breakdown of cell wall or other components due to use of antibiotics. This overt inflammatory response can damage sensitive neurologic tissues. They should not be administered without proper coverage of all infective microorganisms and when the infection is not controlled. Intravitreal dexamethosone in the concentration of 400 microgram in 0.1 ml has been used, but is contraindicated in fungal endophthalmitis [65].

8.3. Pars plana vitrectomy

Although intravitreal antibiotic therapy can provide effective bacterial killing during endophthalmitis, vitrectomy is an appealing adjunct to management. Vitrectomy (surgical cutting and aspiration of vitreous contents and replacement with balanced salt solution) (Figure 6) debrides the vitreous cavity of bacteria, inflammatory cells and other toxic debris; promotes better diffusion of antibiotics; helps in obtaining adequate sampling for microanalysis and helps in speedy recovery of vision [66, 67]. Timing of vitrectomy is controversial, and investigators advocate aggressive early treatment with early vitrectomy in suspected bacterial metastatic endophthalmitis, and more conservative approach in suspected fungal cases. Also,

http://dx.doi.org/10.5772/61608

3 port pars plana 23 or 25 gauge complete vitrectomy is preferred over core vitrectomy. However, in an inflamed eye certain complications like retinal detachment, hypotony and pthisis bulbi can occur. The definite indications for vitrectomy include worsening of signs and symptoms, rapid progression, infections uncontrolled by systemic and /or intravitreal antibiotics, retinal necrosis, extensive subretinal abscess, retinal detachment and intra-ocular foreign body [65].

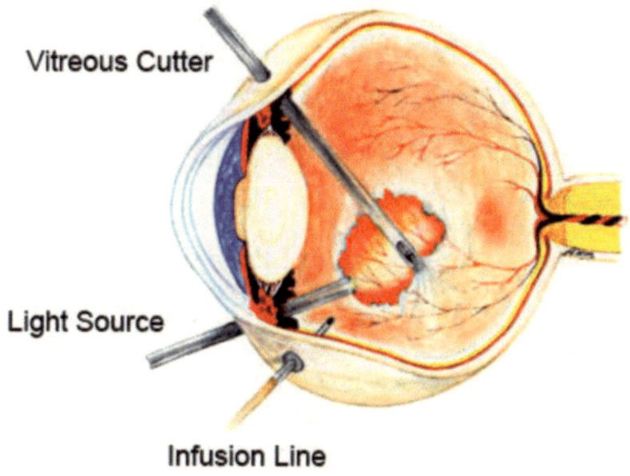

Figure 6. showing Cutting and aspiration of vitreous contents in pars plana vitrectomy

9. Conclusion

Endophthalmitis may cause severe visual loss and detailed understanding of the offending organisms and the intra-ocular host response and its early recognition is necessary for effective treatment of endophthalmitis and improving visual outcome. The key to successful therapy for endophthalmitis is rapid sterilization of the posterior segment by antibiotics and arrest of potentially harmful inflammation, while concurrently limiting risks associated with penetration of the eye by injections or surgery.

Author details

S. Malhotra*, S. Sharma, N. J. K. Bhatia, C. Hans and P. Kumar

*Address all correspondence to: drshalinimalhotra@yahoo.com

Department of Microbiology, Dr. Ram Manohar Lohia Hospital and PGIMER, New Delhi, India

References

[1] Peyman G, Lee P, Seal DV. Endophthalmitis: Diagnosis and Management. Taylor & Francis, London & New York: 2004, pp. 1–278.

[2] Kresloff MS, Castellarin AA, Zarbin MA. Endophthalmitis. Surv Ophthalmol 1998;43:193–224.

[3] Kernt M, Kampik A. Endophthalmitis: pathogenesis, clinical presentation, management, and perspective. Clin Ophthalmol 2010;4:121–35.

[4] Moshfeghi A, Rosenfeld PJ, Flynn HW Jr, et al. Endophthalmitis after intravitreal anti-vascular endothelial growth factor antagonists: a six-year experience at a university referral center. Retina 2011;31:662–8.

[5] Marak Jr GE. Phacoanaphylactic endophthalmitis. Erratum in: Surv Ophthalmol 1992;36:454.

[6] Mamalis N, Edelhauser HF, Dawson DG, Chew J, LeBoyer RM, Werner L. Toxic anterior segment syndrome. J Cataract Refract Surg 2006;32:324–33.

[7] Holland SP, Morck DW, Lee TL. Update on toxic anterior segment syndrome. Curr Opin Ophthalmol 2007;18:4–8.

[8] Carolee M, Cutler P, Jacob B, Sue C, Chris D, Henry EE, Nick M. Toxic anterior segment syndrome: Common causes J Cataract Refractive Surg July 2010;36(7):1073–80.

[9] Stepien KE, Eaton AM, Jaffe GJ, Davis JL, Raja J, Feuer W. Increased incidence of sterile endophthalmitis after intravitreal triamcinolone acetonide in Spring 2006. Retina 2009;29:207–13.

[10] Callegan MC, Engelbert M, Parke DW, Jett BD, Gilmore MS. Bacterial endophthalmitis: epidemiology, therapeutics, and bacterium-host interactions. Clin Microbiol Rev 2002;15:111–24.

[11] Scott IU, Flynn HW, Feuer W, Pflugfelder SC, Alfonso EC, Forster RC, Miller D. Endophthalmitis associated with microbial keratitis. Ophthalmology 1996;103:1864–70.

[12] Krause L, Bechrakis N, Heimann H, Kildal D, Foerster M. Incidence and outcome of endophthalmitis over a 13-year period. Can J Ophthalmol 2009;44:88–94.

[13] Ramakrishnan R, Bharathi M, Shivkumar C, et al. Microbiological profile of culture-proven cases of exogenous and endogenous endophthalmitis: a ten-year retrospective study. Eye (Lond) 2009;23:945–56.

[14] Bahrani HM, Fazelat AA, Thomas M, et al. Endophthalmitis in the era of small gauge transconjunctival sutureless vitrectomy – meta analysis and review of the literature. Semi Ophthalmol 2010;25:275–82.

[15] Akçakaya AA, Sargin F, Erbil HH, et al. A cluster of acute-onset postoperative endophthalmitis over a 1-month period: investigation of an outbreak caused by an uncommon species. Br J Ophthalmol 2011;95:481–4.

[16] Korah S, Braganza A, Jacob P, Balaji V. An "epidemic" of post cataract surgery endophthalmitis by a new organism. Indian J Ophthalmol 2007;55:464–6.

[17] Jamulingam M, Parameswaran SK, Lysa S, Selvaraj M, Madhavan HN. A study on the incidence, microbiological analysis and investigations on the source of infection of postoperative infectious endophthalmitis in a tertiary care ophthalmic hospital: an 8-year study. Indian J Ophthalmol 2010;58:297–302.

[18] Anand AR, Therese KL, Madhavan HN. Spectrum of aetiological agents of postoperative endophthalmitis and antibiotic susceptibility of bacterial isolates. Indian J Ophthalmol 2000;48:123–8.

[19] Peponis V, Rosenberg P, Chalkiadakis SE, Insler M, Amariotakis A. Fungal scleral keratitis and endophthalmitis following pterygium excision. Eur J Ophthalmol. 2009;19:478–80.

[20] Narang S, Gupta A, Gupta V, et al. Fungal endophthalmitis following cataract surgery: clinical presentation, microbiological spectrum, and outcome. Am J Ophthalmol 2001;132:609–17.

[21] Huycke MM, Sahm DF, Gilmore MS. Multiple-drug resistant enterococci: the nature of the problem and an agenda for the future. Emerg Infect Dis 1998;4:239–49.

[22] Forster RK. Etiology and diagnosis of bacterial postoperative endophthalmitis. Ophthalmology Apr 1978;85(4):320-6.

[23] Arshinoff SA, Bastianelli PA. Incidence of postoperative endophthalmitis after immediate sequential bilateral cataract surgery. J Cataract Refract Surg Dec 2011;37(12): 2105–14.

[24] Adán A, Casaroli-Marano RP, Gris O, et al. Pathological findings in the lens capsules and intraocular lens in chronic pseudophakic endophthalmitis: an electron microscopy study. Eye (Lond) 2008;22:113–9.

[25] Al-Mezaine HS, Al-Assiri A, Al-Rajhi AA. Incidence, clinical features, causative organisms, and visual outcomes of delayed-onset pseudophakic endophthalmitis. Eur J Ophthalmol 2009;19:804–11.

[26] Soltau JB, Rothman RF, Budenz DL, Greenfield DS, Feuer W, Liebmann JM, Ritch R. Risk factors for glaucoma filtering bleb infections. Arch. Ophthalmol 2000;118:338–42.

[27] Andreoli CM, Andreoli MT, Kloek CE, Ahuero AE, Vavvas D, Durand ML. Low rate of endophthalmitis in a large series of open globe injuries. Am J Ophthalmol 2009;147:601–8.

[28] Vedantham V, Nirmalan PK, Ramasamy K, Prakash K, Namperumalsamy P. Clinicomicrobiological profile and visual outcomes of post-traumatic endophthalmitis at a tertiary eye care centre in South India. Indian J Ophthalmol 2006;54:5–10.

[29] Gupta A, Srinivasan R, Kaliaperumal S, Saha I. Post-traumatic fungal endophthalmitis—a prospective study. Eye (Lond) 2008;22:13–7.

[30] Callegan MC, Kane ST, Cochran DC, et al. Bacillus endophthalmitis: roles of bacterial toxins and motility during infection. Invest Ophthalmol Vis Sci 2005;46:3233–8.

[31] Romero CF, Rai MK, Lowder CY, and Adal KA. Endogenous endophthalmitis: case report and brief review. Am Fam Phys 1999;60:510–14.

[32] Binder MI, Chua J, Kaiser PK, et al. Endogenous endophthalmitis: an 18-year review of culture- positive cases at a tertiary care center. Medicine 2003;82:97–105.

[33] Ruhnke M, Rickerts V, Cornely OA, et al. Diagnosis and therapy of candida infections: joint recommendations of the German Speaking Mycological Society and the Paul-Ehrlich-Society for Chemotherapy. Mycoses 2011;54:279–310.

[34] Lamaris GA, Esmaeli B, Chamilos G, et al. Fungal endophthalmitis in a tertiary care cancer center: a review of 23 cases. Eur J Clin Microbial Infect Dis 2008;27:343–7.

[35] Safneck JR. Endophthalmitis: a review of recent trends. Saudi J Ophthalmol 2012;26:181–9.

[36] Khan A, Okhravi N, Lightman S. The eye in systemic sepsis. Clin Med 2002;2:444–8.

[37] Lundstrom M, Wejde G, Stenevi U, et al. Endophthalmitis after cataract surgery: a nationwide prospective study evaluating incidence in relation to incision type and location. Ophthalmology 2007;114:866–70.

[38] Behndig A, Montan P, Stenevi U, et al. One million cataract surgeries: Swedish National Cataract Register 1992–2009, J Cat Refract Surg 2011;37:1539–45.

[39] Al-Mezaine HS, Kangave D, Al-Assiri A, Al-Rajhi AA. Acute-onset nosocomial endophthalmitis after cataract surgery: incidence, clinical features, causative organisms, and visual outcomes. Cataract Refract Surg 2009;35:643–9.

[40] Al-Mezaine HS, Al-Assiri A, Al-Rajhi AA. Incidence, clinical features, causative organisms, and visual outcomes of delayed-onset pseudophakic endophthalmitis. Eur J Ophthalmol 2009;19:804–11.

[41] Chaudhry IA, Shamsi FA, Elzaridi E, Al-Rashed W. Al-Amri AM, Al-Anezi F, Arat YO, Holck DEE. Outcome of treated orbital cellulitis from a tertiary eye care center in the Middle East. Ophthalmology 2007;114:345–54.

[42] Cunha-Vaz JG. The blood-ocular barriers: past, present, and future. Doc Ophthalmol 1997;93:149–57.

[43] Steptoe RJ, Holt PG, McMenamin PG. Functional studies of major histocompatibility class II-positive dendritic cells and resident tissue macrophages isolated from the rat iris. Immunology 1995;85:630–7.

[44] Miller KV, Eisley KM, Shanks RM, et al. Recurrent enterococcal endophthalmitis seeded by an intraocular lens biofilm. J Cataract Refract Surg 2011;37:1355–9.

[45] Gilmore MS, Callegan MC, Jett BD. Enterococcus faecalis cytolysin and Bacillus cereus bi- and tri-component toxins. In: Alouf JE, Freer JH. (Eds.) The Comprehensive Sourcebook of Bacterial Protein Toxins, 2nd edn. Academic Press, London, United Kingdom 1999, pp. 419–434.

[46] Projan SJ, Novick RP. The molecular basis of pathogenicity. In: Crossley KB, Archer GL. (Eds.) The Staphylococci in Human Disease. Churchill Livingstone, New York, NY, 1999, pp. 55–82.

[47] Van Snick J. Interleukin-6: an overview. Annu Rev Immunol 1990;8:252–78.

[48] Donahue SP, Kowalski RP, Jewart BH, et al. Vitreous cultures in suspected endophthalmitis: biopsy or vitrectomy? Ophthalmology 1993;100:452.

[49] Spadea L, Fiasca A. Treatment of post-operative endophthalmitis. Eur Ophthal Rev 2012;6(3):149–56.

[50] Joondeph BC, Flynn HW Jr, Miller D, et al. A new culture method for infectious endophthalmitis. Arch Ophthalmol 1989;107:1334.

[51] Dworkin LL, Gibler TM, Van Gelder RN: Real-time quantitative polymerase chain reaction diagnosis of infectious posterior uveitis. Arch Ophthalmol 2002;120:1534–9.

[52] Wittwer CT, Kusukawa N: Real-time PCR. In: Persing DH. (Ed.) Molecular Microbiology: Diagnostic Principles and Practice. Washington, DC: ASM Press, 2004, pp. 71–84.

[53] Results of the Endophthalmitis Vitrectomy Study. A randomized trial of immediate vitrectomy and of intravenous antibiotics for the treatment of postoperative bacterial endophthalmitis. Endophthalmitis Vitrectomy Study Group, Arch Ophthalmol 1995;113:1479–96.

[54] Chan IM, Jalkh AE, Trempe CL, Tolentino FI. Ultrasonographic findings in endophthalmitis. Ann Ophthalmol Aug 1984;16(8):778–84.

[55] Alp BN, Elibol O, Sargon MF, et al. The effect of povidone iodine on the corneal endothelium. Cornea 2000;19:546–50.

[56] ESCRS Endophthalmitis Study Group: Prophylaxis of postoperative endophthalmitis following cataract surgery: results of the ESCRS multi-centre study and identification of risk factors. J Cataract Refract Surg 2007;33:978–88.

[57] Liu SJ, Kau YC, Liaw CW, Peng YJ. In vitro elution of vancomycin/amikacin/ steroid from solvent-free biodegradable scleral plugs. Int J Pharm 2009;370:75–80.

[58] Peng YJ, Kau YC, Wen CW, Liu SJ. Solvent-free biodegradable scleral plugs providing sustained release of vancomycin, amikacin, and dexamethasone—an *in vivo* study. J Biomed Mater Res Part A 2010;94:426–32.

[59] Nelson ML, Tennant MTS, Sivalingam A, et al. Infectious and presumed noninfectious endophthalmitis after intravitreal triamcinolone acetonide injection. Retina 2003;23:686–91.

[60] Wiechens B, Neumann D, Grammer JB, Pleyer U, Hedderich J, Duncker GI. Retinal toxicity of liposome-incorporated and free ofloxacin after intravitreal injection in rabbit eyes. Int Ophthalmol 1998–1999;22:133–43.

[61] Foster RE, Martinez JA, Murray TG, Rubsamen PE, Flynn HW, Forster RK. Useful visual outcomes after treatment of Bacillus cereus endophthalmitis. Ophthalmology 1996;103:390–7.

[62] Ferencz JR, Assia EI, Diamantstein L, Rubinstein E. Vancomycin concentration in the vitreous after intravenous and intravitreal administration for postoperative endophthalmitis. Arch Ophthalmol 1999;117:1023–7.

[63] Ferencz JR, Assia EI, Diamantstein L, Rubinstein E, Vancomycin concentration in the vitreous after intravenous and intravitreal administration for postoperative endophthalmitis. Arch Ophthalmol 1999;117:1023–7.

[64] Recchia FM, Busbee BG, Pearlman RB, Carvalho-Recchia CA, Ho AC. Changing trends in the microbiologic aspects of postcataract endophthalmitis. Arch Ophthalmol 2005;123:341–6.

[65] Lamaris GA, Esmaeli B, Chamilos G, et al. Fungal endophthalmitis in a tertiary care cancer center: a review of 23 cases. Eur J Clin Microbiol Infect Dis 2008;27:343–7.

[66] Mathews AS, Pillai GS, Natasha R, Shetty M. Endogenous endophthalmitis – a review. Kerala J Ophthalmol 2011;23:25–31.

[67] Fujii GY, De Juan E Jr, Humayun MS, et al. Initial experience using the transconjunctival sutureless vitrectomy system for vitreoretinal surgery. Ophthalmol 2002;109:1814–20.

[68] Fine HF, Iranmanesh R, Iturralde D, Spaid RF. Outcomes of 77 consecutive cases of 23-gauge transconjunctival vitrectomy surgery for posterior segment disease. Ophthalmol 2007; 114:1197–200.

Chapter 3

Ocular Parasitic Infections – An Overview

Nancy Malla and Kapil Goyal

Additional information is available at the end of the chapter

http://dx.doi.org/10.5772/64137

Abstract

Eyes are said to be the windows of body, by which this beautiful world is visualized. Human eye has a unique structure and is vulnerable to numerous infections. Whenever anatomical structures are breached, host defenses come into play, but if infection is severe and not treated timely, it could lead to visual impairment or blindness. Parasitic infections are considered, the significant causes of ophthalmic diseases worldwide. In this chapter, an overview of ocular parasitic infections (OPI) is detailed out, with an initial brief introduction followed by description of anatomy of the human eye and various defense mechanisms to provide better understanding of the parasitic infections affecting different parts of human eye. The last part includes individual details of various human ocular parasitic infections.

Ocular infections can be classified based on either the etiological agent or according to the anatomical site of infection. The parasitic etiological agents include mainly protozoa, helminths and ectoparasites. Due to the complex life cycles of parasites and their tendency to cause wide range of pathologic lesions, different parasites/parasitic infections have been addressed separately, including brief epidemiology, clinical features, diagnosis and treatment.

Keywords: Eye, parasitic infections, protozoa, nematodes, cestodes, trematodes, ectoparasites

1. Introduction

The ocular parasitic infections (OPI) are considered significant causes of ocular pathologies worldwide [1]. The common protozoal parasites primarily infecting the ocular tissue(s) are *Acanthamoeba* species and *Toxoplasma gondii* [2–7]. In addition, case studies of eye diseases caused by *Leishmania, Trypanosoma cruzi, Entamoeba histolytica, Hartmannella, Plasmodium falciparum, Microsporidia* and *Giardia lamblia* have been rarely reported [1, 8, 9]. Among the helminths, ocular infections are caused primarily by nematode parasites (*Onchocerca volvulus,*

Loa loa, Toxocara canis and Toxocara cati) [1, 8, 10–12]. In addition, case studies of ocular infections caused by other nematodes (*Angiostrongylus cantonensis, Dirofilaria repens, Trichinella spiralis, Thelazia callipaeda, Baylisascaris procyonis, Wuchereria bancrofti* and *B. malayi*), cestodes (*T.solium cysticercus, Echinococcus granulosus*, and *Multiceps multiceps* larvae) and trematodes (*Fasciola hepatica and Schistosoma* species) have been reported from different geographical areas [1, 8, 13–15]. The ectoparasites infecting the eye include larvae of flies [16] (*Oestrus ovis, Rhinoestrus purpureus, Dermatobia hominis, Chrysomia bezziana, Lucilia* spp., *Cuterebra, Hypoderma, Cochliomyia, Wohlfahrtia, Gastrophilus*), *Phthirus pubis*, hard and soft ticks (belonging to class Arachnida) [1, 17]. Ocular pentastomiasis caused by the larval stage of Pentastomida, the crustacean-related parasites, is reported to cause permanent loss of vision due to the retinal detachment or lens subluxation [18]. Further, with the advent of HIV/AIDS (human immunodeficiency virus/acquired immune deficiency syndrome), few ocular infections have also been reported in HIV-infected patients [19, 20].

Ocular parasitic infections have been widely reported from different geographical areas (Table 1), mainly depending on the endemicity of the parasite(s). The prevalence depends primarily on the geographical distribution of the parasite, socioeconomic environment and immune status of the patient. The common modes of infection are direct contact (blepharoconjunctivitis caused by *Leishmania, Acanthamoeba* keratitis, microsporidial infections, infestation caused by lice and mites) [21–23], through blood stream (Toxoplasma chorioretinitis, retinal involvement in malaria, uveitis caused by *Toxocara*) [1, 23, 24], congenital transmission (Toxoplasmosis) and zoonotic transmission (primarily infectious diseases of animals that can naturally be transmitted to humans) [25]. In addition, few of the helminths that may lead to ocular infection are transmitted by vectors (onchocerciasis, dirofilariasis and thelaziasis), consumption of contaminated food (sparganosis, trichinellosis) and indirectly from the environment (fascioliasis, ascariasis and echinococcosis).

Adult and/or larval stages of the parasites may reside in human ocular tissues externally or in the ocular globe. The clinical symptoms and signs vary, depending on the etiological agent and the ocular tissue/part involved. However, local defense mechanisms and host immune responses play role in establishing the infection. The pathology in the eye can occur due to direct damage by the infecting pathogen, indirectly by toxic products, immune mediated or ectopic localization by ectoparasites. The clinical diagnosis usually mimics other pathologies due to numerous etiologies both infectious and non-infectious, which can cause conjunctivitis, keratitis, uveitis and endopthalmitis [26]. Thus, a high index of clinician suspicion is required for infective parasite etiology in patients having inflammation in the eye. In addition, eye can be involved in various systemic disorders and thorough ocular examination along with history of travel to the endemic area, risk factors and other associated medical illness that help in establishing the preliminary diagnosis. However, confirmatory diagnosis is usually achieved by direct demonstration of parasite in clinical samples and/or pathological changes observed by either slit lamp or biopsy examination [1, 8, 27, 28]. The antigen and antibody detection in ocular fluids and/or serum usually substantiates the clinical diagnosis in few parasitic infections (Toxoplasmosis, malaria, leishmaniasis, ocular gnathostomiasis, cysticercosis, toxocariasis, echinococcosis) [1, 10, 29, 30]. Molecular techniques including detection of parasite DNA by polymerase chain reaction (PCR) have added new dimensions in the diagnosis and species identification [31–36]. The treatment of choice is mostly surgical excision,

http://dx.doi.org/10.5772/64137

while in few infections, medical treatment is usually advised either in conjunction with surgical procedure (onchocerciasis, dirofilariasis [37], cysticercosis [38], echinococcosis [39], myiasis, infections due to ticks and mites) or for inoperable patients. Although surgical excision is usually reserved for worms that are large, it is also recommended for space-occupying lesions of the orbit. Drug resistance is posing problem for the effective medical treatment, thus necessitating the discovery of new antiparasitic drugs [32]. Prevention and control measures differ in various infections and usually include proper health education and awareness of various risk factors. The various experimental animal models for few of the ocular infections have been successfully established to study the pathogenic mechanisms, drug efficacy and local immune responses [40, 41].

Although issues mainly are the timely diagnosis and treatment, yet many challenges need to be considered/addressed.

2. Anatomy

Diagrammatic representation of human eye depicting significant ocular parasitic infections is shown in Figure 1.

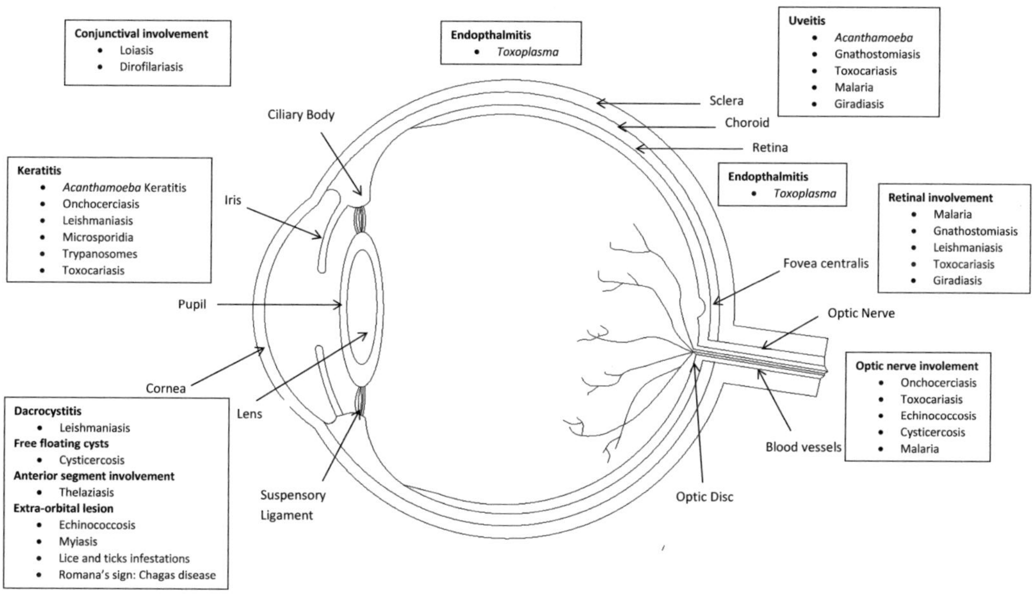

Figure 1. Human eye anatomy depicting significant ocular parasitic infections.

2.1. Orbits

The eye balls along with extraocular muscles, nerves, blood vessels and fat are situated in the bony cavities known as orbits. The periosteal covering of the bony orbit fuses with orbital septum and duramater. Abscess due to infectious agent can localize in the space beneath the periostium. The paranasal sinuses are separated from it by the floor, medial wall and roof of the orbit and may act as the source of orbital infection. Lamina papyracea are the thinnest bony walls, which separate orbit from ethmoidal sinuses. Thus, any breach in it causes the ingress of sinus microbiota to orbital tissue leading to infection. Orbital cellulitis can also be caused by direct extension of the infection from the ethmoidal sinuses to the orbital cavity. The lateral wall of the sphenoidal sinus constitutes the medial wall of the optic canal and infection of the former can percolate to the latter causing optic nerve damage and visual loss. There are various apertures present in the orbital cavity, which provides the route of communication with the adjacent structures. The superior and inferior orbital fissures, the lacrimal fossa, nasolacrimal duct and the optic canal constitute such important apertures [1, 42–46].

2.2. Blood supply

The ophthalmic artery and its branches constitute main arterial supply of orbit. The majority of the venous drainage occurs through superior ophthalmic vein, which drains into cavernous sinus that is located just posterior to the orbital apex. Veins from the facial region and many anterior ophthalmic veins anastomose and drain into cavernous sinus through superior orbital vein. Thus, cavernous sinus is prone to infection from facial region and also from the orbital region through the superior ophthalmic vein leading to a serious complication.

2.3. Eyelids

The eyelids impart two protective anatomical barriers, i.e., orbital septum and conjunctiva. Former divides the orbit from the eyelid into preseptal and postseptal spaces and provides a physical barrier to infectious agents and latter one is reflected back on itself, which provides protection by hindering the free movement of the material posteriorly from the anterior surface of the globe.

2.4. Lacrimal system

Lacrimal system consists of lacrimal gland, accessory gland and excretory system. Tears are secreted by lacrimal gland, which flows over the cornea and finally drain into nasal cavity by nasolacrimal duct through lacrimal sac. Any obstruction to the nasolacrimal duct can lead to regurgitation of the accumulated fluid onto the ocular surface leading to increased chances of infection.

2.5. Layers of eye ball

The basic structure of eye ball or globe consists of three concentric layers. The outermost covering is composed of sclera and cornea. The middle covering is composed of uveal tract, consisting of choroid, ciliary body and iris. The inner most covering is retina. The sclera is almost avascular except for the presence of superficial small blood vessels. The choroid is a highly vascular structure and provides nutrition and oxygenation to the retina beneath it. Due

http://dx.doi.org/10.5772/64137

to these qualities, choroid serves as a fertile area for the proliferation of various pathogens, which spread by hematogenous route.

2.6. Anterior and posterior chambers

Anterior segment of the eye in front of the vitreous humor comprises anterior one-third of the eye and is further divided into anterior chamber and posterior chamber. Anterior chamber is the space between posterior surface of cornea and the iris, whereas posterior chamber is the space between iris and the front of vitreous. The aqueous humor is produced by non-pigmented ciliary epithelium in the posterior chamber and drains through the pupillary aperture into the anterior chamber. Cornea is composed of well-organized collagen fibrils, which is avascular in nature. Lens is also an avascular crystalline structure, which continues to grow throughout life. Thus, aqueous humor fills these spaces and provides nutrition to the surrounding structures.

2.7. Vitreous humor

It is a gel-like substance present in front of retina and posterior to the lens in the posterior segment of the eye. It is optically clear and is composed of collagen framework interspersed with hyaluronic acid. During intraocular inflammation, it becomes hazy and may cause impairment of vision.

2.8. Retina and optic nerve

Retina constitutes the innermost covering of the eye ball and captures the light energy with the help of rods and cones. The outer half of the retina is supplied by central retinal artery, whereas inner half receives its blood supply from the choroid.

The optic nerve is formed by axons of the inner cell layer that exits the globe. It is covered by all the three meningeal coverings, which are direct extensions of the brain coverings. Thus, it is vulnerable to infections originating from both within cranial vault and within orbits.

3. Ocular defense mechanisms

The surface of the eye is well protected by both mechanical and immunological defense mechanisms. To breach the defense mechanism, some form of trauma is essential. The eyelids provide mechanical protection to the surface of eyeball. The eyelashes protect against airborne particles and trauma by initiating blink reflex. The cornea is also sensitive to tactile sensation and helps in the initiation of blink reflex, which is provided by dense sensory nerve endings. The lids direct the tears, particulate debris, allergens and microbes to the lacrimal excretory system by its sweeping action over the anterior surface of the eyeball. Bell's phenomenon also provides protection to cornea as globe is turned upwards and slightly outwards during eyelid closure to avoid corneal exposure [47]. Meibomian glands secrete lipids, which provide stability to the tear film. The epithelial surface of the cornea and conjunctiva provides anatomical barrier to the pathogens. This function is further strengthened by the impermeability provided by the basement and cellular junctional complexes of the cornea. Indigenous flora of the eye also provides protection by creating a competition for colonization by the pathogens.

Immune defense mechanisms are provided by the vascular supply of the eye. Any breach in the anatomical defense system initiates the ocular inflammatory response, which helps in vasodilation and exudation of immunologically active substances and cells [1, 8, 48–52].

3.1. Defenses of the tear film

There are three layers of the tear film: oil, aqueous and mucous. Majority of the tear film is composed of aqueous layer and pH of the tear film helps in neutralization of toxic substances. Flow of tears help in mechanical flushing of the foreign particles and allergens into the lacrimal excretory system. Mucosal layer helps in entrapment of pathogens. Tear film contains various immunological active substances such as lactoferrin, lysozyme, β-lysin, ceruloplasmin, complement and immunoglobulins.

3.2. Conjunctival defenses

The conjunctival associated lymphoid tissue lies beneath the conjunctiva. It consists of both B and T lymphocytes. B and T cell precursors mature when exposed to foreign particles or allergens, then migrate to regional lymph nodes for further development, and thereafter return to the conjunctiva through blood stream to produce specific immunoglobulins and cellular defense responses.

3.3. Corneal defenses

Although the cornea is avascular, it is provided by limited defense mechanisms in the form of Langerhans cells (dendritic cells) and immunoglobulins. The surface of the cornea is covered by mucous glycoprotein, which helps in cross-linkage of the IgA and protects the anterior surface of the cornea. Immune defense mechanisms are activated whenever injury occurs, leading to recruitment of the polymorphonuclear cells, lymphocytes and fibroblasts.

3.4. Cellular immune responses

Langerhans cells are situated along the peripheral margin of the cornea and conjunctiva. These cells possess receptors, which help in phagocytosis and processing of certain antigens for presentation. Langerhans cells stimulate B and T cells to elicit a strong cellular immune response. During inflammation Langerhans cells migrate toward the cornea, causing increased release of inflammatory substances.

3.5. Leukocyte defense

Polymorphonuclear leukocytes are the hallmark of acute inflammation and are associated with oxygen-dependent pathways for the generation of free radicals that help in killing of the invading pathogens. Another immune defense mechanism operated by the production of defensins is antimicrobial proteins active against wide range of pathogens.

3.6. Defensins

Ocular surface is constantly exposed to environment and foreign bodies, thus there are greater chances of infection. However, robust innate immune system at ocular surface protects the eye from infection. There are several peptides of defensins and cathelicidin families that are present in tear film and secreted by corneal and conjunctival cells. These are not only antimicrobial in nature but also help in the recruitment of immune cells and thus provide a link to adaptive immunity. The important defensins present in human eye are hBD-1 (human beta defensins), hBD-2, hBD-3, CAP37 (Cathelicidin-related antimicrobial peptide), LL37 (type of cathelicidin) and HNP-1, 2, 3 (human neutrophil defensins) [53].

4. Protozoan eye infections

4.1. Toxoplasmosis

Toxoplasmosis is caused by obligatory intracellular protozoan parasite known as *Toxoplasma gondii.* The mode of infection is either by the ingestion of oocysts shed in feces of the cats or other Felidae (definitive host) or by the consumption of tissue cyst present in the raw or uncooked meat. Life cycle of *Toxoplasma* includes three stages that are oocysts, tachyzoites and bradyzoites. It completes its life cycle in two phases, one as an intestinal phase in its homologous host, such as cats and another as an extraintestinal phase in its heterologous host, such as mouse, man and other animals. When cats feed on mouse brain containing tissue cysts of *T. gondii,* a large number of oocysts are released in the infected cat's feces. After 1–5 days, oocysts get matured and become infective to man and other animals. After ingestion, oocysts liberate sporozoites, which penetrate intestinal mucosa and reach to distant organs such as brain, eyes, liver, spleen, lymph nodes, heart, skeletal muscles and placenta by blood and lymphatic stream. *Toxoplasma* tissue cysts also occur in the skeletal muscles of the intermediate host such as sheep and pigs (Figure 2) [54]. In addition, developing fetus can acquire the infection transplacentally from the mother during pregnancy. Rarely, infection may also result from consumption of drinking water contaminated with oocysts. The ocular infection can be either congenital or acquired.

Approximately, one-third of the world's population is thought to be infected by *T. gondii.* It is common in hot and humid climates such as Central America, Asia and the Caribbean region (Table 1, Figure 3). In Europe, toxoplasmosis is common and the highest prevalence rates have been reported in France. Various risk factors such as geographical region, meat consumption, personal habits, animal reservoir and climatic conditions play a significant role in the transmission of infection. In recent years, due to indoor keeping of livestock and improvement in hygiene standards, the risk of acquiring infection has decreased tremendously in the developed nations. However, in the developing nations, risk has increased due to population growth, urbanization trends and increase in meat consumption. Drinking water, seawater and

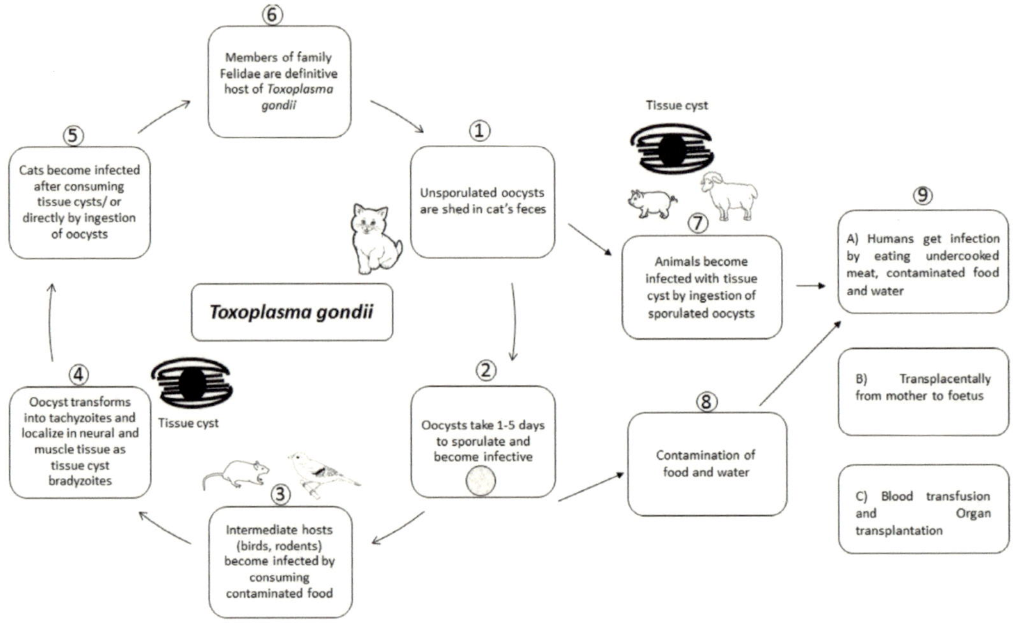

Figure 2. Life cycle of *T. gondii* (Diagrammatic representation).

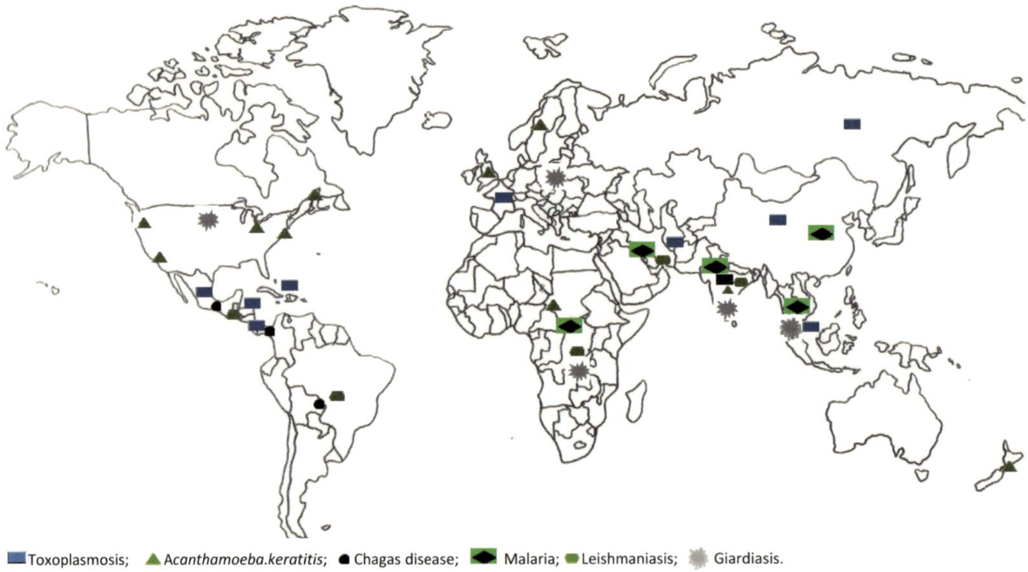

Figure 3. World map showing geographical areas endemic for ocular protozoal infections.

seafood contaminated with oocysts when consumed may account for many unreported cases. Therefore, exact prevalence would be much higher than reported in the literature [55–58].

Ocular toxoplasmosis usually manifests in immunocompromised *T. gondii*-infected individuals and in neonates who acquire infection transplacentally [4]. The main target organs in congenital toxoplasmosis are the brain, eyes and placenta. *T. gondii* disseminates through the blood stream, lodges at particular site(s) and develops into tissue cysts. The dendritic cells and macrophages act as "Trojan horses" to guide the parasite through blood-brain barrier to reach at its target site in brain [59]. Inside the host cell, it protects itself from the toxic host molecules by hiding inside the parasitophorous vacuole (structure produced by apicomplexan parasites that allows the parasite to develop inside host cell and protects from phagolysosomes). There are three main clonal lineages of *T. gondii.* Type I strains being the highest virulent, whereas types II and III are moderately virulent. However, at present more than 130 "atypical" genotypes are known, but their exact role in pathogenesis is not well established. Host genetic factors such as polymorphism in Toll-like receptors (TLR) (TLR2, 5 and 9) are also known to play a role in the susceptibility to and severity of ocular toxoplasmosis [60, 61].

Congenital ocular toxoplasmosis usually involves both the eyes, whereas acquired ocular toxoplasmosis is usually unilateral [62, 63]. Chorioretinitis is caused by necrotizing inflammation due to the rupture of an older cyst. Intense form of chiretinitis may occur in newborns and patients infected with HIV. In addition, congenital toxoplasmosis patients may present with wide range of ocular symptoms such as strabismus, nystagmus and blindness. Acute, acquired infection may result in photophobia, scotoma and loss of central vision. Ptosis may occur due to oculomotor nerve involvement.

Diagnosis of ocular toxoplasmosis in children with congenital infection is established by recognizing distinctive clinical findings such as focal necrotizing retinitis, vitritis, anterior uveitis and cataract [64] However, in cases with atypical presentation or having severe fulminant disease, diagnosis is usually established by analyzing the intraocular fluid for the presence of specific antibodies or the presence of parasite DNA by molecular techniques such as PCR or real-time PCR [65, 66]. PCR is performed by targeting the *Toxoplasma* B1 gene or other multiple repeat sequences [67–69]. Though, in general, PCR with amniotic fluid is known to have significantly high sensitivity (64%) and specificity (100%) for the diagnosis of toxoplasmosis [70], sensitivity of only 53 and 83% has been documented for the diagnosis of ocular toxoplasmosis [71]. PCR can be performed on either aqueous humor or vitreous fluid, but aqueous humor can be collected more easily. However, the DNA burden in aqueous humor is low, and in rare instances a confirmation would necessitate vitreous sampling [72].

Antibody detection in serum samples is widely used for establishing the diagnosis of toxoplasmosis [73–76], while its role is limited in establishing the diagnosis of the ocular toxoplasmosis. A rising titer of specific IgG over a period of 3 weeks helps in establishing the diagnosis [77]. The detection of specific antibodies in intraocular fluids by the enzyme-linked immunosorbent assay (ELISA) is the most commonly used test for the diagnosis of toxoplasmosis. The Goldmann-Witmer coefficient (GWC) calculation is a common method to estimate the local versus systemic *Toxoplasma*-specific IgG. This index helps in measuring the intraocular levels of specific antibodies against *Toxoplasma*. It is expressed as the level of *Toxoplasma*-specific IgG relative to the level of total IgG in the aqueous humor as a fraction of the level of *Toxoplasma*-specific IgG relative to the level of the total IgG in the serum. A value of 2 or above is considered as an evidence of intraocular infection. Toxoplasma specific IgG antibodies are produced in response to the actively multiplying tachyzoites at local site of infection [72, 78] The presence of *T. gondii*-specific IgM is the hallmark of a recently acquired systemic or, possibly, ocular infection. However, high rate of false-positive results due to the persistence of antibodies, decreases its utility as a diagnostic marker for recent ocular toxoplasmosis. In patients with reactivated ocular toxoplasmosis, it is not useful as *T. gondii*-specific IgM antibodies are either absent or present in very low quantity [79]. Saliva samples have also been tested for the detection of specific antibodies for the diagnosis of toxoplasma encephalitis in immunocompromised individuals, but it may play a limited role in ocular toxoplasmosis [74].

An algorithm for the laboratory confirmation of clinically suspected cases of ocular toxoplasmosis has been reported [72]. Reactivated form of ocular toxoplasmosis is considered in patients with typical lesions of toxoplasmic retinochoroiditis, specific IgG seropositive, specific IgM seronegative and responding to anti-*Toxoplasma* treatment. However, if patients are specific IgM seropositive, then additional laboratory tests are required. If doubt persists about diagnosis, paired serum and aqueous samples are required to be tested in parallel. The clinical diagnosis along with laboratory evidence is documented in 60-85% of cases and thus, laboratory evidence is lacking in 15-40% of clinically suspected patients. Analysis of aqueous humor is useful in patients presenting with atypical ocular lesions or not responding to specific treatment [72].

In immunocompetent individuals, toxoplasma retinochoroiditis usually resolves within 2–3 months [80]. Classic therapy or triple therapy with a combination of pyrimethamine, sulfadiazine and systemic corticosteroids is recommended for lesions involving or near to fovea, an area critical for vision. Classic therapy is usually associated with significant side effects, therefore other drugs such as trimethoprim-sulfamethoxazole, clindamycin, atovaquone and azithromycin are being evaluated for the treatment of ocular toxoplasmosis [81].

Trimethoprim-sulfamethoxazole (Bactrim) appears to be a safe and effective substitute for sulfadiazine, pyrimethamine and folinic acid for the treatment of ocular toxoplasmosis.

Progressive and recurring necrotizing retinitis, with vision-threatening complications such as retinal detachment, choroidal neovascularization and glaucoma, may occur at any time during the clinical course if the infection is not treated on time. Congenital toxoplasmosis can lead to cataract. The aim of the treatment is to arrest parasite multiplication during the active period of retinochoroiditis and to minimize damage to the retina and optic disc [64].

Animal model(s) can be used to study various aspects of ocular toxoplasmosis [40].

4.2. *Acanthamoeba* keratitis

Acanthamoeba keratitis (AK) is caused by *Acanthamoeba* spp., a free-living protest parasite [82]. The word "acanth" in Greek means "spikes" and has been added as a prefix to "amoeba" to denote the spine-like structures present on its surface. The parasite is present ubiquitously in the environment and exists in two forms, trophozoite and cyst forms. In humans, it can enter through eye, nasal passage or ulcerated broken skin (Figure 4). Infection of the eye can cause blinding keratitis and life-threatening granulomatous encephalitis. Various risk factors contributing to the development of *AK* are (1) wearing of contact lenses for long time, (2) poor personal hygiene, (3) cleaning of lenses with contaminated water and (4) formation of biofilm on contact lenses [82].

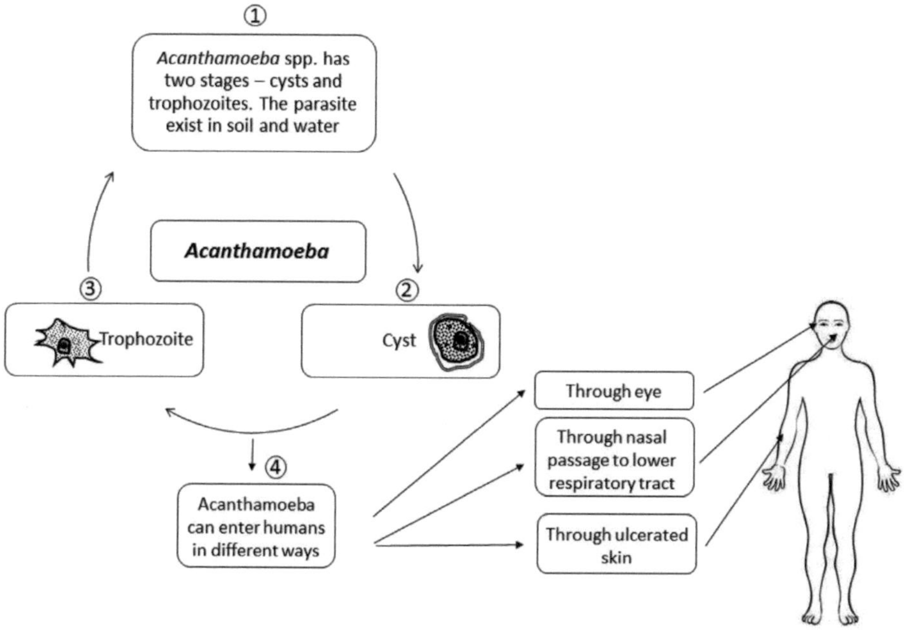

Figure 4. Life cycle of *Acanthamoeba* (Diagrammatic representation).

Acanthamoeba keratitis is common among the contact lens users, and its geographic distribution is depicted in Table 1 and Figure 3. However, in India the infection is reported even in non-contact lens users [7]. The incidence of *Acanthamoeba* keratitis in developed nations varies from 1 to 33 cases per million contact lens wearers. In developing nations where contact lens users are limited, the other suggested risk factors are trauma, exposure to contaminated water, use of traditional eye medicine, low socioeconomic background, splashing contaminated water into the eye following dust fall and corneal injury with mud [7, 22, 83]. The pathogenesis of *Acanthamoeba* involves following sequential events, i.e., breach in the epithelial barrier, invasion of stroma by amoeba, depletion of keratocytes, induction of inflammatory response, photophobia and finally necrosis of stroma leading to blindness [82].

The diagnosis of AK is difficult as it is usually confused with symptoms of bacterial, fungal or viral keratitis. However, history of contact lens use together with a history of excruciating pain is a strong indication toward the diagnosis of AK. For establishing the clinical diagnosis with high sensitivity, in vivo confocal microscopy can be used, which is a non-invasive procedure. The *Acanthamoeba* cysts appear as hyper-reflective, spherical structures that are well defined because of their double wall. However, trophozoites are difficult to distinguish from leukocytes and keratocyte nuclei [84, 85]. Laboratory confirmation is established by direct demon-

Ocular protozoal infections	Geographical distribution
Toxoplasmosis	Worldwide particularly in Central America, Asia, Caribbean region, Europe particularly in France
Acanthamoeba keratitis	Worldwide significantly in Chicago, San Francisco, Boston, Philadelphia, Sweden, Portland, New Zealand, United Kingdom, India, Africa
Chagas disease	Central and South America
Malaria	Africa, Central & South America, Middle East and Asia
Leishmaniasis	Africa, Mediterranean region, Middle East, Central and South America, parts of Asia
Microsporidiosis	Worldwide
Giardiasis	Southeast Asia, South Africa, Europe and USA
Ocular nematode infections	
Onchocerciasis	Africa, South America, Arabian peninsula
Loiasis	Central and West Africa
Dirofilariasis	Asia, Africa and Europe
Gnathostomiasis	South East Asia particularly Thailand, China, Japan and India, Central and South America particularly in Mexico, Guatemala, Peru and Ecuador
Thelaziasis	Asia Pacific region - China, India, Thailand, Indonesia, Japan and Korea
Toxocariasis	Worldwide particularly in Asia, Japan, Korea, Ireland, Alabama
Ocular cestode infections	
Cysticercosis	Indian subcontinent, Central and South America, Africa and Far East
Echinococcosis	South America, Middle East, Mediterranean countries, India and Australia
Ocular trematode infections	
Fascioliasis	France, Spain, Italy, Austria, Belgium, United Kingdom, Algeria, Tunisia, Iran, Uzbekistan, Korea, China, Argentina, Chile, Peru, Brazil, Guatemala
Schistosomiasis	Sub-Saharan Africa, China, South Asia
Philopthalmosis	Europe (Yugoslavia), Israel, Asia (Thailand, India, Sri Lanka, Japan) and America (i.e., Mexico, and the United States)
Clinostomum lacramalitis	Thailand
Fascioliasis	Iran
Alaria mesocercariasis	San Francisco, California
Ocular infections by ectoparasites	
Myiasis	Worldwide with greater abundance in poor socioeconomic regions of tropical and subtropical countries, Mediterranean basin and Middle East
Phthiriasis palpebrum	Case reports from Tunisia, Taiwan, India, Pakistan, China, Korea, Lebanon, Israel, Brazil, Turkey, United Kingdom, Belgium, Italy, Cyprus, United States of America (USA)
Tick infestation	Case reports from Ireland, Turkey and USA

Table 1. Ocular parasitic infections and geographical distribution

stration of parasite by immunofluorescence microscopy or by isolating the parasite in culture. Although culture remains the gold standard, it is tedious and time consuming. Multiplex real-time PCR assays (multiplex assays targets more than one region and simultaneously can detect two or more target regions) have also been developed for the detection of different pathogenic free-living amoeba and/or different genotypes of *Acanthamoeba*. Although molecular techniques have high sensitivity and specificity, these are only available at apex laboratories and also require a well-established molecular laboratory [86]. Newer techniques such as Matrix-Assisted Laser Desorption Ionization Time-Of-Flight (MALDI-TOF) and ^{1}H-NMR spectroscopy [87] are also being tested for the rapid identification of *Acanthamoeba* in the clinical specimens [88].

Chances of recovery are good if the pathogen is restricted to cornea epithelium but can lead to vision loss, if it invades stroma leading to necrosis and intense inflammation. Medical treatment, if started early, can lead to a significant improvement within 2–3 weeks [89].

Preventive measures include thorough and adequate disinfection of contact lenses. It is recommended to remove contact lenses before any activity involving contact with water, including showering, using a hot tub, or swimming. Hands should be washed with soap and water and dried before handling contact lenses. Contact lenses should not be rinsed with tap water and should be cleaned and stored as per manufacturer's guidelines. It is suggested that the increased awareness about the other predisposing factors (corneal injury, fall of foreign body in eye) among the general public may enable early and frequent recognition and proper management of AK in patients other than contact lens wearers [7].

4.3. Chagas disease

Chagas disease or American trypanosomiasis is caused by *Trypanosoma cruzi* [90]. It is a chronic systemic disease, included in the WHO's list of most neglected tropical diseases. Approximately, 8 million people are known to be affected in Latin America (Table 1, Figure 3) [8]. The life cycle of the parasite is passed in two stages involving trypomastigotes and amastigotes forms as depicted briefly in Figure 5. *T. cruzi* passes its life cycle in two hosts: one in man or the reservoir host and other in the transmitting insect. The infection is transmitted by the blood-sucking triatomine bugs when infective metacyclic trypomastigotes in bug's feces are released onto the skin of humans. These infective trypomastigotes enter the human host when bite wound is either scratched or rubbed, or through permissive mucosal or conjunctival surfaces. Parasites circulate in the human body affecting various tissues and organs. If the initial bite of the triatomine bug is near the orbit, it may lead to severe palpebral and periorbital edema (Romana's sign) [91]. It causes a painless edema and constitutional symptoms of fever, malaise and anorexia are common. Ocular involvement (posterior uveitis) in congenital Chagas disease is recently reported. Although ocular fundus examination has been unobtrusive, small parafoveolar retinal pigment epithelium defects have been reported in 7.6% of chagasic patients [92].

The diagnosis of acute Chagas disease is established by the direct demonstration of trypomastigotes in the blood/buffy coat preparation. Parasites can also be isolated by direct culturing of blood on NNN medium (Novy, MacNeal, Nicolle's medium). It may take 7 to 10 days for culture to become positive. Diagnosis may also be established by xenodiagnosis. During acute phase, the role of serology is limited in the diagnosis as antibodies take time to

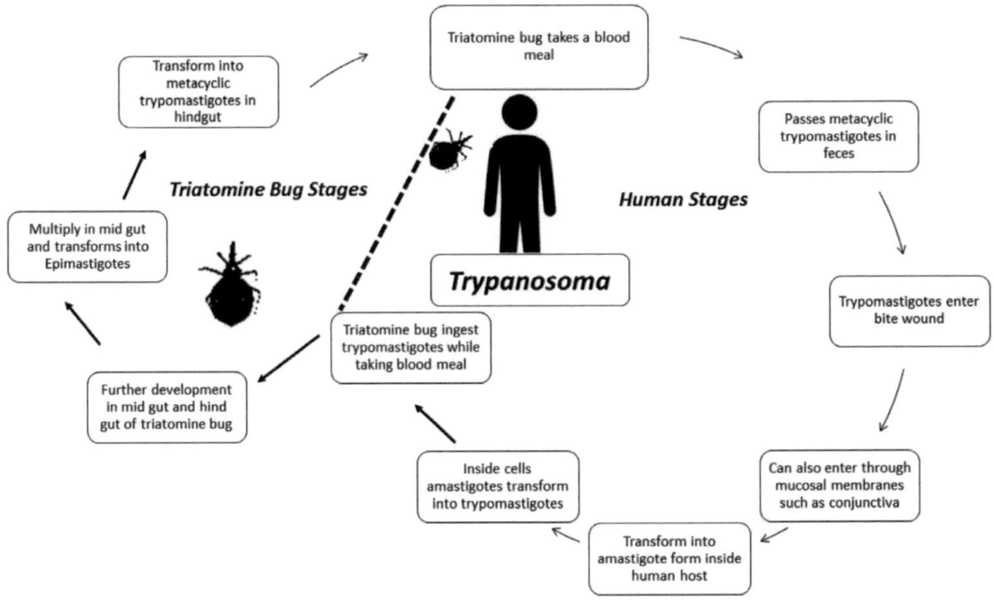

Figure 5. Life cycle of *Trypanosoma cruzi* (Diagrammatic representation).

develop and false positive results have also been known to be associated with serological tests due to cross-reaction of antibodies to non-pathogenic *Trypanosoma rangeli* [8, 91]. Furthermore, detailed examination by the ophthalmologist may aid in establishing the diagnosis. However, accumulation of retinal pigment epithelium defects have been shown in patients with intraocular involvement of intermediate and chronic Chagas disease in Paraguay/South America, but overall fundus examination has shown to be unobtrusive [92, 93].

Acute cases of Chagas disease are treated by nifurtimox and benznidazole. Benznidazole is given as 5–7.5 mg/kg per day orally in two divided doses for 60 days. Nifurtimox is given as 8–10 mg/kg per day orally in three or four divided doses for 90 days [91, 94].

Within few weeks, symptoms of acute Chagas disease such as Romana's sign fade away, but infection persists. The average life-time risk of developing complications of chronic phase is around 30%. It may take more than 20 years to develop chronic complications. However, trypanocidal therapy did not significantly reduce cardiac clinical deterioration through 5 years of follow-up as documented by randomized trial of benznidazole for chronic Chagas' cardiomyopathy [95, 96].

4.4. Leishmaniasis

Leishmaniasis is caused by protozoan parasite that belongs to genus *Leishmania.* Humans get infection by the bite of phlebotomine sand flies. There are different clinical forms of leishmaniasis, such as visceral leishmaniasis (VL), cutaneous, diffuse cutaneous and mucocutaneous caused by different species of *Leishmania.* Worldwide, approximately 1.3 million new cases occur every year with a mortality of 20,000 to 30,000 persons per annum [97]. While taking the blood meal, infected sandfly injects promastigotes into humans. Further in the human body, the promastigotes are transformed into amastigote forms, and these are engulfed by tissue macrophages. Amastigote forms replicate inside the cells and further spread either systemically or through cutaneous route, depending on the species of the parasite (Figure 6). Ocular involvement due to leishmaniasis has been reported from various countries such as India, Sudan, Italy, Norway, Turkey and Iran (Table 1, Figure 3) [98–103]. Anterior uveitis is the most common ocular manifestation in VL, which can occur during the course of infection and can further progress to glaucoma [104, 105]. Focal retinal whitening, cotton wool spots, hemorrhages and increased vessel tortuosity have also been reported on fundus examination [106–110]. In severe cases, flame-shaped lesions also appear, which denote hemorrhage from the anterior capillaries of the nerve fiber layer. These findings have also been correlated with anemia and thrombocytopenia as these hemorrhages usually get resolved with treatment, leading to improvement in anemia/thrombocytopenia. Optic neuropathy has been reported due to mucosal leishmaniasis. Eyelid involvement has been documented in cutaneous and mucocutaneous leishmaniasis [111, 112]. Severe involvement can progress to ptosis and ectropion secondary to cutaneous leishmaniasis leading to keratopathy and altered vision [112]. However, eyelid is rarely involved by leishmaniasis and is reported in approximately only 2.5% of cases with cutaneous leishmaniasis [113]. The most common aspect of eyelid leishmaniasis is chalazion-like lesions, but other forms such as ulcerous, phagedenic, cancer-like forms and unilateral chronic granulomatous blepharitis may be observed. Chronic dacryocystitis has been reported in patients suffering from mucocutaneous leishmaniasis, which can effect formation of tear film, leading to dryness of eyes [114]. Endo-ocular lesions have been observed in patients having disseminated cutaneous leishmaniasis. A report from Brazil documented the presence of *Leishmania* in the aqueous humor along with iridiocyclitis [115]. Although ocular manifestations are not very common, it is suggested that a person with ocular manifestation from endemic country should undergo fundus examination for early diagnosis [116].

Diagnosis of leishmaniasis can be achieved by the direct demonstration of parasites in the tissue smears and/or biopsy samples, culture technique(s), antigen and/or antibody detection and molecular technique(s). However, each technique has its own merits and demerits. Amastigotes can be easily identified in the cutaneous and mucocutaneous lesions but are not easily identified in cases with ocular disease [103, 117, 118]. Molecular techniques such as PCR/real-time PCR can identify the genome of parasite with greater sensitivity (100%) and specificity (100%) [119, 120]. The treatment of leishmaniasis depends on several factors such as clinical form of the disease. The antileishmanial drugs include pentavalent antimony, sodium stibogluconate, liposomal Amphotericin B, miltefosine and paromomycin [118, 121].

Ocular lesions do not heal without treatment and could lead to vision loss if conjunctiva is involved due to severe ulceration. Healing occurs without visual impairment if treatment is initiated early during the course of infection and vigorous treatment is required to prevent blindness [121, 122].

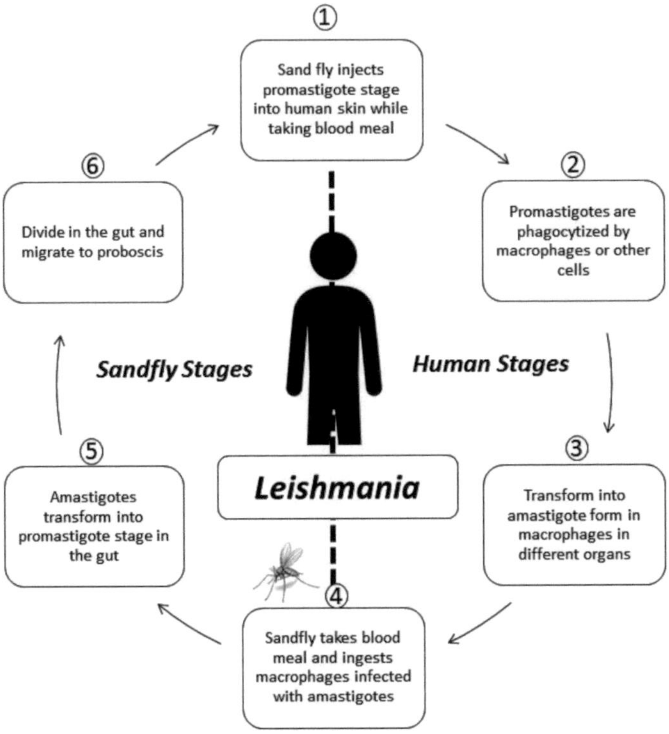

Figure 6. Life cycle of *Leishmania* (Diagrammatic representation).

4.5. Malaria

Malaria is caused by the parasites of Genus *Plasmodium* and is transmitted by the bite of female anopheles mosquitoes. The malarial parasite passes its life cycle in humans and mosquitoes. Inside human host, *Plasmodium* undergoes exoerythrocytic and erythrocytic schizogony as shown briefly in Figure 7. Malarial parasite multiplies by asexual method (schizogony) while residing inside liver cell and the red blood cells. After the parasites have undergone erythrocytic schizogony for a certain period, some of the merozoites give rise to gametocytes, which are taken up by mosquitoes during their blood meal. The gametocytes further develop into sporozoites that are infective to man. Sporozoites when introduced into humans are not directly infective for red blood cells, but undergo development initially in hepatic cells (exoerythrocytic schizogony) and later on invade red blood cells to complete erythrocytic schizogony. As per World Malaria Report 2014 [123], an estimated 3.3 billion people are at risk of developing malaria (Table 1, Figure 3). Complications of severe malaria due to *P. falciparum* mainly occur due to the sequestration of malarial parasite in the microvasculature leading to occlusion and hypoxia. Most of the ocular manifestations occurring in malaria are a result of the same mechanism. Sequestration is further amplified by auto agglutination and resetting [124, 125].

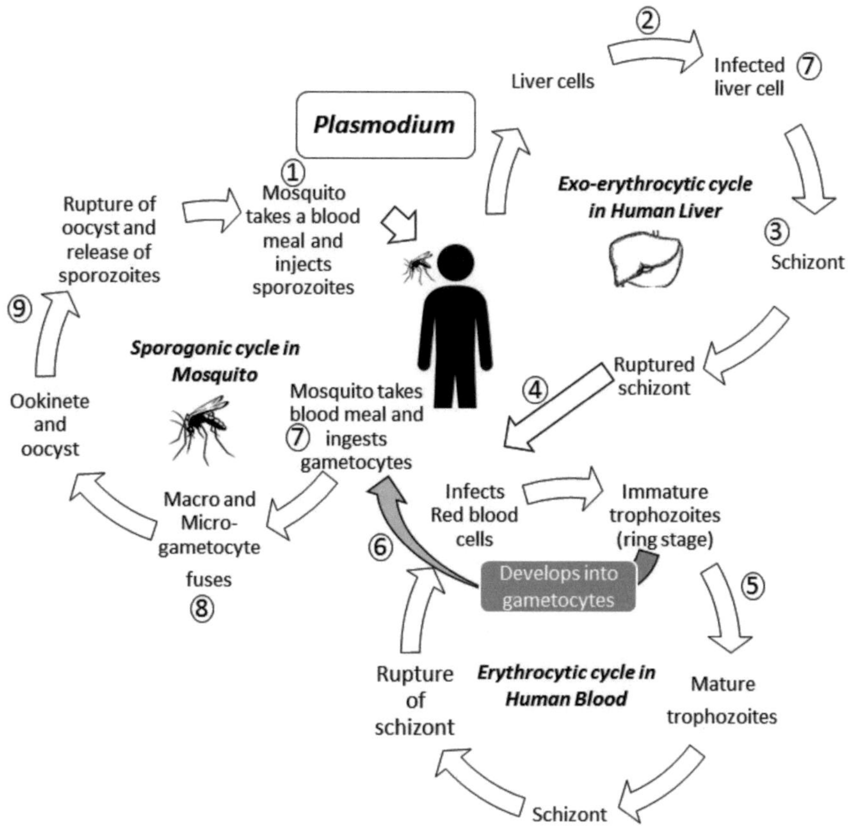

Figure 7. Life cycle of *Plasmodium* (Diagrammatic representation).

Wide range of ocular symptoms has been reported in patients suffering from malaria. Uncomplicated malaria is usually not associated with significant ocular findings but rarely may be associated with edema and hyperemia of the eyelids, chemosis of conjunctiva, conjunctival hemorrhage and anterior uveitis [126]. On the other hand, severe ocular manifestations may occur in cerebral malaria due to *P. falciparum* leading to visual field defects, cortical blindness, optic neuritis, papilledema and optic atrophy [127]. Ocular motor disturbances have also been reported. Occasionally, infarcts in brainstem may cause changes in pupillary reaction and disorders of eye movements. Patients with cerebellar syndromes may present as nystagmus [128, 129]. Characteristics features such as retinal whitening consisting of irregular patchy areas may be localized or diffused in all segments of retina [130]. Blood vessel changes manifest as discoloration (white or orange) occurring mainly in the peripheral fundus, whereas white-centered retinal hemorrhages may manifest as malaria retinopathy. Discoloration of retinal vessels occurs due to the absence of hemoglobin in parasitized erythrocytes, sequestered within retinal vasculature and thus cannot reflect normal red color. Retinal changes in cerebral malaria are considered as poor prognostic markers [131]. The prevalence of any retinopathy, papilledema, hemorrhages, vessel changes, macular whitening and peripheral whitening has been reported in 61, 15, 46, 32, 46 and 44%, respectively, among children with cerebral malaria in Malawi [132].

Diagnosis of malaria is established by light microscopy or by rapid antigen detection kits. Light microscopic examination of Giemsa-stained peripheral blood smear is considered as gold standard for the diagnosis of malaria with a threshold of about 50–100 parasites/μL [133]. However, in addition, ocular examination may provide clue to the diagnosis as specific retinal changes can be seen directly [129, 134, 135].

Treatment depends on the species of *Plasmodium* causing infection. Artemisinin combination therapy is recommended for malaria due to *P. falciparum*. Artemisinin combination therapy includes short-acting artemisinin derivative and long-acting antimalarial (sulphadoxine-pyrimethamine, lumefantrine). Chloroquine along with primaquine is recommended for malaria due to *P. vivax*. Ocular toxicity [136] is very well documented with chloroquine therapy. This includes corneal changes (cornea verticillata) and corneal deposits. Toxic maculopathy and scotoma has also been reported. Quinine overdose has also been known to cause decreased vision, retinal and macular degeneration, mild scotomas and color vision defects [136].

If not treated, malarial retinopathy is associated with serious consequences as reports indicate that the severity of retinopathy is related to prolonged death and coma. After antimalarial treatment and resolution of coma in severe malaria, malarial retinopathy resolves after some time [132, 137].

4.6. Microsporidiosis

Microsporidiosis is the term used to denote the infection caused by microsporidia belonging to phylum Microspora [23]. Microsporidia were once thought to be protists but are now known to be fungi. Although it is classified as a protozoal disease in ICD-10, their phylogenetic placement has been resolved to be within the fungi [138]. Microsporidiosis is considered as an opportunistic infection in AIDS/HIV-infected individuals and is prevalent worldwide (Table 1) [1]. Microsporidia are small, unicellular, spore forming, obligate intracellular pathogens. Important genera responsible for ocular manifestations are Encephalitozoon and Nosema. Another species, Septata, has also been reported to cause keratoconjunctivitis [139]. The prevalence of microsporidiosis ranges from 2 to 50% among severely immunocompromised, HIV-infected patients found in North America, western Europe and Australia. The prevalence data for microsporidiosis is limited among non-HIV-infected persons [9].

1. The life cycle of parasite involves three stages (Figure 8):
2. The resistant spore (infective form)
3. The spore injects the infective sporoplasm into the host cell. Inside the host cell, sporoplasm undergoes multiplication either in the cell cytoplasm or inside parasitophorous vacuole. Microsporidia develop to mature spores by sporogony that are released by disruption of cell membrane. The free mature spores are the infective forms.

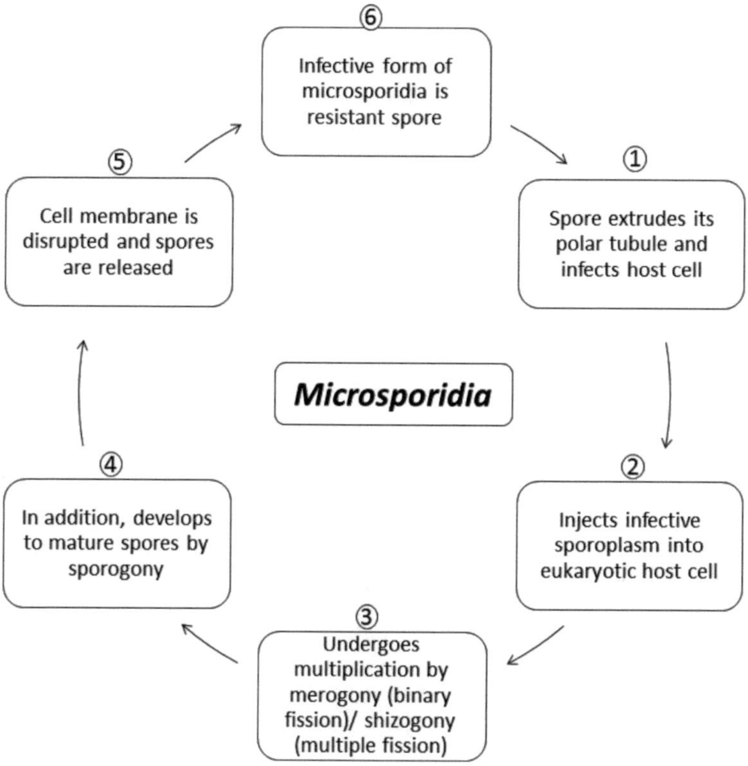

Figure 8. Life cycle of *Microsporidia* (Diagrammatic representation).

Ocular manifestations caused by *Microsporidia* are mainly limited to conjunctiva and cornea. Corneal involvement may lead to punctate epithelial keratitis, hyphema, necrotizing keratitis and corneal ulcer. Symptoms include foreign body sensation, photophobia and decrease in visual acuity [23].

Diagnosis is established by direct demonstration of the spores by microscopy or electron microscopy of the corneal scrapping or biopsy specimens. Isolation of the parasites in culture has also been attempted [140]. There are no reports on use of serological tests to detect antibodies in serum or tears in ocular microsporidiosis [9]. Lesions usually heal after 1–2 weeks as it is self-limiting. Treatment of microsporidial keratoconjunctivitis with polyhexamethylene biguanide does not offer any significant advantage but treatment with topical fumagillin showed significant improvement [141–143].

4.7. Giardiasis

Giardiasis is caused by *Giardia duodenalis* (syn. *G. lamblia* or *G. intestinalis*) [144]. The infection is transmitted by ingestion of contaminated water/food or directly by feco-oral route. The parasite exists in trophozoite and cyst forms as shown in Figure 9. In the trophozoite stage the parasite multiplies in the intestine of man by binary fission. When conditions become unfavorable in the small intestine, encystment occurs and cysts are released along with feces. After ingestion, within 30 minutes, cyst hatches out trophozoites that further multiply in the small intestine. It is found both in developing and developed nations (Table 1, Figure 3). Although it mainly causes diarrhea and malabsorption, in one-third of the patients, it can also result in long-term extra intestinal manifestations [145].

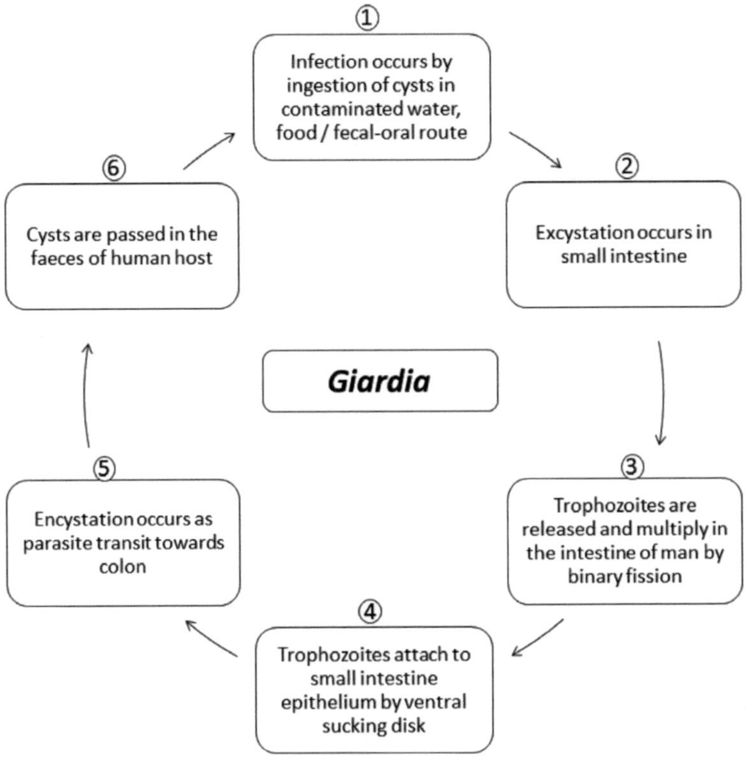

Figure 9. Life cycle of *Giardia lamblia* (Diagrammatic representation).

Barraquer was the first to report the ocular manifestation (iridiocyclitis, choroiditis and retinal hemorrhages) in patients who were suffering from diarrhea due to *G. duodenalis.* Retinal changes in the form of "salt and pepper" degeneration have been reported in children suffering from giardiasis. Corsi et al. [146] reported salt and pepper retinal changes in 19.9% of the patients with giardiasis. This occurs due to the damage of the retinal cells and subsequent release of pigment granules in retina giving an appearance of blackish dots on a background of light yellow pink retina. The exact mechanism(s) by which giardiasis leads to ocular manifestations is still unknown, although possibility of direct invasion by the parasite is excluded (137). Further studies are desired to exactly pinpoint the mechanism by which retinal manifestations follow the occurrence of intestinal giardiasis. Alterations in the retinal pigment layer are most common but do not cause functional changes in retina, and these lesions do not progress or regress with time [146].

http://dx.doi.org/10.5772/64137

The diagnosis is established by direct demonstration of the parasite in the fecal samples by microscopy. Concentration techniques of the samples yield higher sensitivity. Nitroimidazole group of drugs are highly effective against *G. duodenalis*. Most commonly used drugs are metronidazole for 5–7 days or ornidazole/tinidazole in single dose [147]. Treatment of intestinal infection is recommended if present, but no specific treatment is required for ocular manifestations related to retina [146].

5. Nematode infections

5.1. Onchocerciasis

Onchocerciasis, also known as "river blindness", is caused by *Onchocerca volvulus*, the filarial nematode. It is transmitted from person-to-person by the repeated bites of infected blackflies (*Simulium* species). These blackflies are mostly found near the flowing rivers and streams and transmit the infection to the people residing in nearby remote villages [148]. The life cycle of the parasite passes between black flies and humans as shown in Figure 10. While taking a blood meal, stage 3 larvae present in infected blackfly are transmitted onto human skin and penetrate into bite wound. In subcutaneous tissue, these larvae develop into adult filariae. Adult worm produces hundreds of thousands of embryonic larvae (microfilariae) that may persist for 3-5 years in the human host. These embryonic larvae migrate to the skin, eyes and other organs. The microfilariae are ingested by the female blackfly when it bites infected humans and develop further in the blackfly. During subsequent bites, it transmits infection to new human host [148, 149].

Onchocerciasis mainly occurs in tropical countries and majority of the cases (99%) have been reported from sub-Saharan Africa. It is also found in some countries of the Middle East and Latin America such as Brazil, Guatemala, Mexico and Venezuela (Table 1, Figure 11). Approximately, 25 million people are known to be affected by onchocerciasis worldwide, and it is known to cause visual impairment and blindness in approximately 800,000 and 300,000 people, respectively [148, 150]. The inflammatory response initiated against dying microfilariae causes gradual and progressive loss of vision due to sclerosal keratitis [149, 151]. Apart from causing keratitis, clinical features may also manifest as iridiocyclitis, chorioretinitis and optic atrophy. Autoimmune mechanisms have also been postulated to cause inflammation in the posterior eye. Accumulation of retinal and retinoic acids, strong eosinophilic response and immune reaction against *Wolbachia* antigens [152] released by dying microfilariae also contributes to the ocular pathogenesis [153].

The filarial parasites of major medical importance in humans contain the symbiotic bacterium *Wolbachia,* and reports have revealed that targeting of these bacteria with antibiotics results in a reduction in worm viability, development, embryogenesis and survival. *Wolbachia* is present as an intracellular bacteria symbiont in all the developmental stages of *Onchocerca volvulus.* Clearance of the endosymbionts by antibiotic treatment causes inhibition of worm development. *Wolbachia* contributes directly to the metabolic activity of the nematode. Various

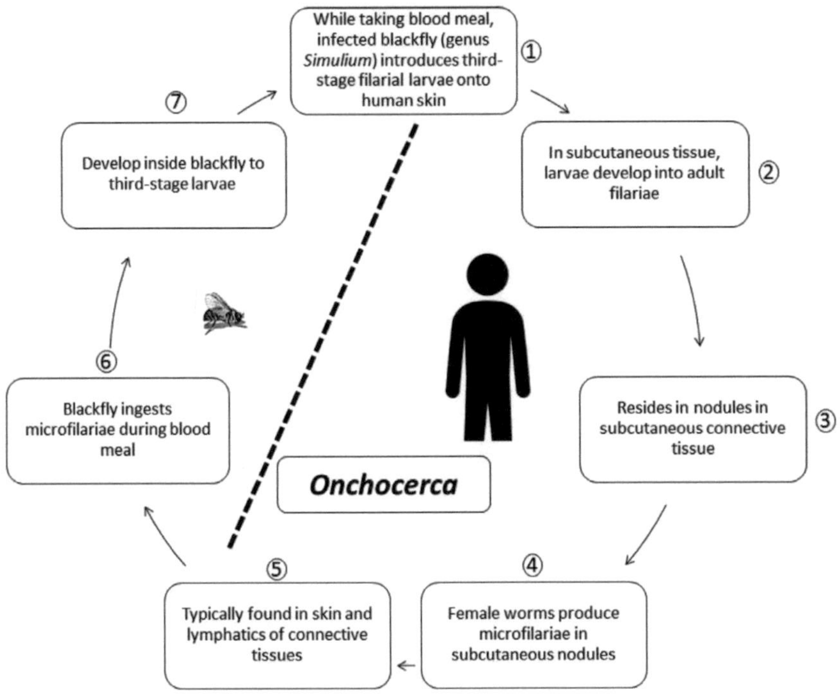

Figure 10. Life cycle of *Onchocerca volvulus* (Diagrammatic representation).

biochemical pathways such as heme, nucleotide and enzyme co-factor biosynthesis are intact in *Wolbachia* but absent or incomplete in nematode [154].

Diagnosis is difficult to establish in light infections. Skin snips can be subjected to microscopy for visualizing the larvae, but it yields very low sensitivity. Infections of the eye can be diagnosed with direct demonstration of the parasite by slit-lamp examination or by demonstrating the parasite in sclerocorneal punch biopsy. Newer techniques such as skin-snip PCR can establish the diagnosis if larvae are not visualized [155]. Antibodies can be detected by ELISA or EIA, but these tests cannot distinguish between past and current infections [156, 157]. Skin-snip PCR has 84–91% sensitivity and 100% specificity [149]. The sensitivity and specificity of serum antibody detection has been reported to be 78–99% and 95–100%, respectively [149]. A promising antigen detection by dipstick assay was recently developed, but its specificity was found to be low in high endemic areas due to cross reaction with urine filarial antigen [158, 159]. Xenodiagnosis (exposing possible infected tissue to a vector and then examining the vector for the presence of microorganism) has also provided clue in some cases.

If the infection is not treated on time, it can progress toward blindness [160]. Drug of choice for the treatment is ivermectin, given 150 to 200 μg /kg body weight, every 6 months to prevent the skin damage and blindness. Treatment with ivermectin has been shown to decrease visual field loss and severity of keratitis. Ivermectin only kills the larvae but not the adult worms. Doxycycline can be used to kill the adult worm. The mechanism of action is that it kills the

http://dx.doi.org/10.5772/64137

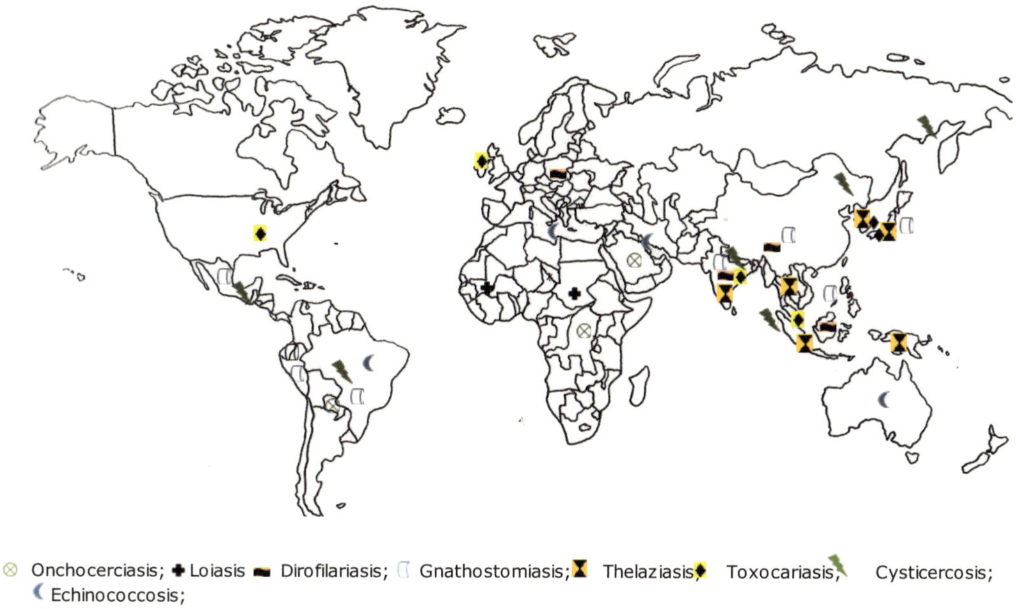

Figure 11. World map showing geographical areas endemic for ocular nematode and cestode infections.

Wolbachia bacteria residing in the worm, on which the adult worm depends for its survival. Treatment with a 6-week course of doxycycline has been shown to kill more than 60% of adult female worms and to sterilize 80–90% of females 20 months after treatment. Thus, treatment with ivermectin is advised one week prior to treatment with doxycycline to provide relief to patient [148, 161].

The best method to get the protection from insect bite is the use of insect repellent. Community-directed treatment with ivermectin (CDTI) along with vector control measures is the main approach to control onchocerciasis. Ivermectin kills microfilariae and also prevents adult worms from producing more microfilariae for few months following treatment, so reduces transmission [148].

5.2. Loiasis

Loiasis is caused by *Loa loa*, the African eyeworm. It is transmitted by the bite of tabanid flies, belonging to the genus *Chrysops*. It affects approximately 3 million people, residing in certain rain forests of Central and West Africa (Table 1, Figure 11) [162, 163]. The tabanid flies most commonly bite during day time and are more common during rainy season. The smoke of wood fires and movement of people attract them. These flies are more commonly found near rubber plantations and are attracted by the well-lit homes. The larvae are passed from flies to humans when humans are bitten by these flies [162]. The larvae develop into adults in the human host over one year and migrate through cutaneous and subcutaneous tissue (Figure 12). Migration of the adult worm is painless, but it is associated with mild tingling sensation. It may involve the nasal area, bulbar conjunctiva and eyelids [164].

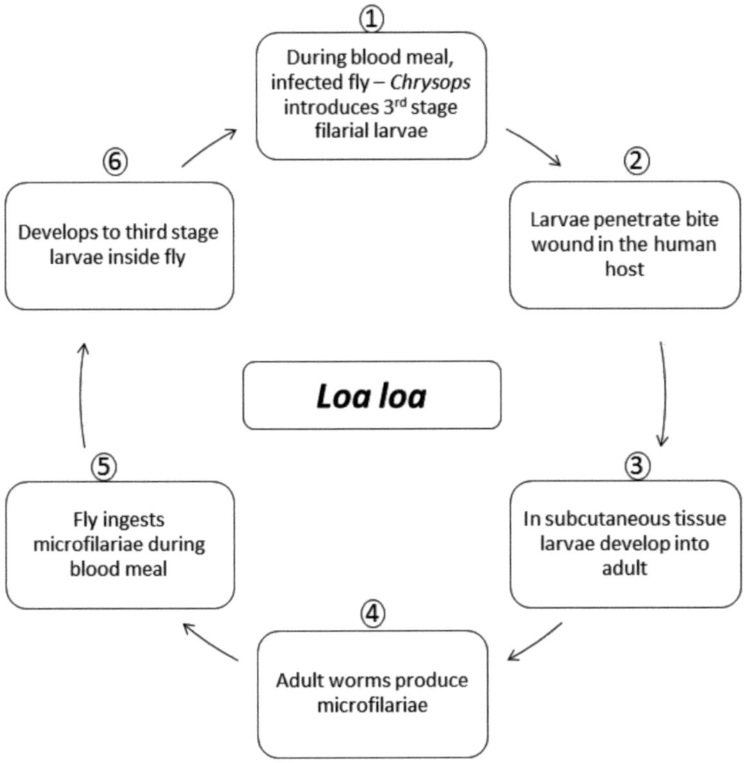

Figure 12. Life cycle of *Loa loa* (Diagrammatic representation).

Ocular manifestations may occur due to the presence of both microfilariae and adult worms. The adult worms may survive up to 15 years and have been found in the conjunctiva, vitreous, eyelid and anterior chamber. Calabar swellings [165] may occur as a result of localized angioedema due to intense atopic reaction. Retinal hemorrhages may occur due to aneurysmal dilatation of the retinal vessels due to the invasion of the retinal and choroid vessels by the microfilariae present in blood stream. Perivascular inflammation can also be present, and ocular examination under slit lamp examination is useful in establishing the diagnosis.

The diagnosis is usually confirmed by the direct demonstration of the microfilariae in the blood by visualizing Giemsa-stained slides under the microscope. However, many of the individuals having visible worm in the eye may test as amicrofilaraemic [166]. Blood should be drawn during the midday as this time coincides with the periodicity of the microfilariae in the blood. The microfilariae can also be demonstrated in unstained blood smear. Adult worm extraction establishes the diagnosis in patients having conjunctival involvement [167]. Antibody detection [168] may aid in establishing the diagnosis, but its presence cannot differentiate between recent and past infection. Eosinophilia and high IgE also indicate active infection [169].

Eye worm if not treated causes very little damage to eye as it lasts less than one week (often just hours). Surgical removal relieves eye symptoms, in addition medical treatment is required

http://dx.doi.org/10.5772/64137

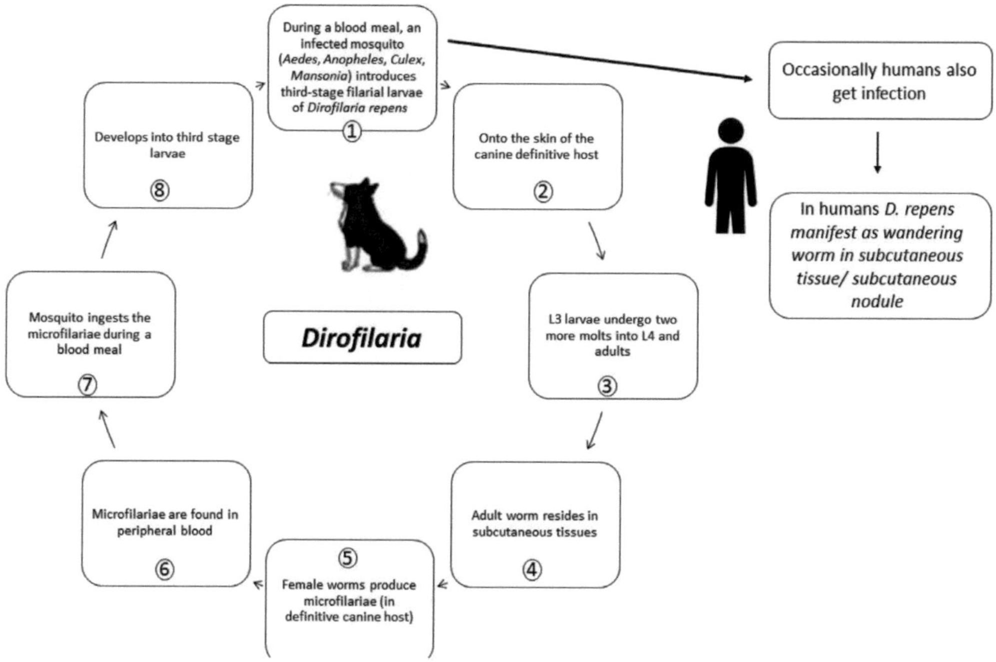

Figure 13. Life cycle of *Dirofilaria repens* (Diagrammatic representation).

for treating loiasis [170]. Therapy involves manual removal of adult worms and administration of diethylcarbamazine (DEC), which kills both adult worms and microfilariae.

5.3. Dirofilariasis

Dirofilariasis is caused by nematodes belonging to the genus *Dirofilaria.* The various species of *Dirofilaria* that are natural parasites of domestic and wild animals are *D. immitis, D. repens, D. tenuis* and *D. ursi* [37]. It is prevalent worldwide and is an important zoonotic infection. It is being reported in increasing numbers from Mediterranean countries such as Italy and have also been reported from France, Greece, Spain, Croatia, India, Serbia, Denmark, Russia and Tunisia (Table 1, Figure 11). The parasite passes its life cycle in canids as definitive host as shown in Figure 13. Mosquitoes act as intermediate host and vector for the transmission of infection from animals to human host. Mosquitoes take up microfilariae along with blood meal from the infected host, develop inside the mosquitoes and are subsequently transmitted to other hosts while taking a fresh blood meal. Larvae migrate from the subcutaneous tissue to the right side of the heart and/or to other parts of the body where maturation takes place. Depending on the site of lodgment, it can cause pulmonary, cardiovascular, subcutaneous or ocular infection [28].

There are several cases that document ocular involvement due to dirofilariasis [37, 171–173]. Ocular symptoms depend on the site of infection. Eyelid involvement [174] leads to edema, pain, pruritus and congestion of conjunctiva, whereas intraocular [175] involvement leads to foreign body sensation, diplopia, photophobia and floaters.

Diagnosis can be established by the direct demonstration and identification of the adult worm. Intraocular presence of the parasite can be confirmed by ophthalmoscopy. Serological techniques are not useful in establishing the diagnosis due to the cross reaction with other parasitic helminths, particularly *Toxocara canis*. Recombinant proteins proved to exhibit 100% sensitivity and 90% specificity by ELISA for the diagnosis of pulmonary dirofilariasis [176].

Without treatment, worm remains in eye causing symptoms due to its presence [177]. Surgical excision is the treatment of choice; however use of diethylcarbamazine (DEC) has also been reported with some success [37, 178].

5.4. Gnathostomiasis

Gnathostomiasis is a food-borne zoonotic parasitic infection, caused by ingestion of raw or undercooked freshwater fish, pork, chicken, frog and snake [179, 180] contaminated with the third-stage larvae of *Gnathostoma* species. The life cycle of the parasite passes in pigs, cats and wild animals as definitive host, whereas small crustaceans act as first intermediate host and fish, frog or snake act as second intermediate host as depicted in Figure 14. In the infected person, larvae migrate through viscera and reach internal organs and subcutaneous tissues. Depending on the location of lodgment, it can cause cutaneous, visceral, ocular or cerebral gnathostomiasis. Majority of the cases have been reported from East Asia (Thailand, China, Japan and India) and Central and South America (Mexico, Guatemala, Peru and Ecuador) (Table 1, Figure 11). However, sporadic cases have been reported worldwide [181]. *Gnathostoma spinigerum* is the most common species causing infection in humans.

Ocular manifestations occur due to the migration of the parasite and its metabolites, leading to inflammatory response. Conjunctiva and corneal infection may lead to congestion of the conjunctiva and corneal ulceration, respectively. Intraocular involvement may lead to glaucoma, uveitis, retinitis and vitreous hemorrhage [182, 183]. In severe cases, retinal detachment has also been reported due to the fibrinous scarring along the migratory path.

Diagnosis is difficult to establish and high index of suspicion is required. Patients may present with marked eosinophilia [184] and elevated IgE levels [185]. ELISA for specific antibody detection and histopathological examination of the biopsy samples may assist in establishing the diagnosis [186–188]. ELISA for antibody detection reported to have low sensitivity, ranging from 59 to 87%, with a specificity of 79–96% [189, 190]. If parasite is not removed, it leads to persistence of visual disturbances such as floaters. Surgical treatment is curative and only modality available [191].

5.5. Thelaziasis

Thelaziasis is caused by nematode *Thelazia callipaeda*, transmitted to humans by drosophilid flies [192]. It is also known as oriental eyeworm due to its geographical distribution in Asia Pacific region (China, India, Thailand, Indonesia, Japan and Korea) and Russia [12, 193] (Table

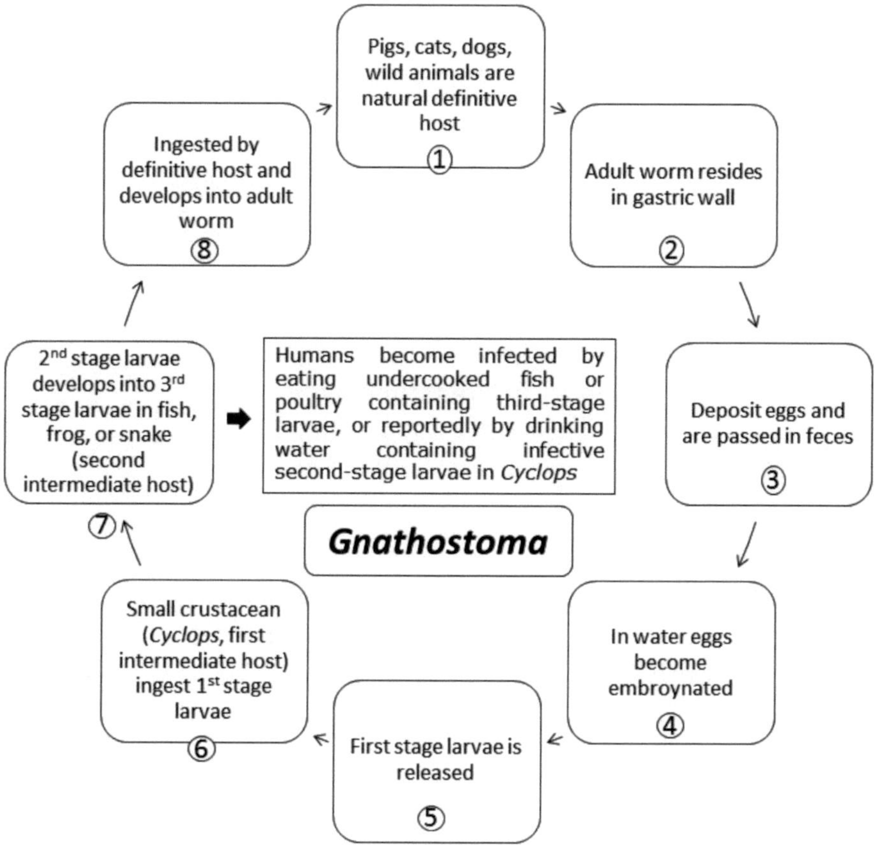

Figure 14. Life cycle of *Gnathostoma* (Diagrammatic representation).

1, Figure 11). The life cycle passes in dogs and other canids, cattle and horses as definitive host and flies act as intermediate host as shown in Figure 15. First-stage larvae are present in the lacrimal secretions of infected humans/animals. The arthropod vectors while feeding on infected lacrimal secretions ingest these larvae, which further develop into infective third-stage larvae. The vector transmits accidentally third-stage larvae when it feeds on lacrimal secretion of other persons/animals. Within 5–6 weeks, these larvae further develop into adult form in the eye of an infected person. These parasites mainly cause infection of the anterior segment of the eye, but intraocular infections involving vitreous and retina have also been reported. It is a disease associated with poor personal hygiene.

Without treatment, worm remains in eye causing symptoms due to its presence [194]. Treatment is surgical removal of worms along with the topical application of thiabendazole. Preventive measures include use of bed nets at night, maintenance of personal hygiene and keeping surroundings clean to control the vector population responsible for the transmission of infection [8].

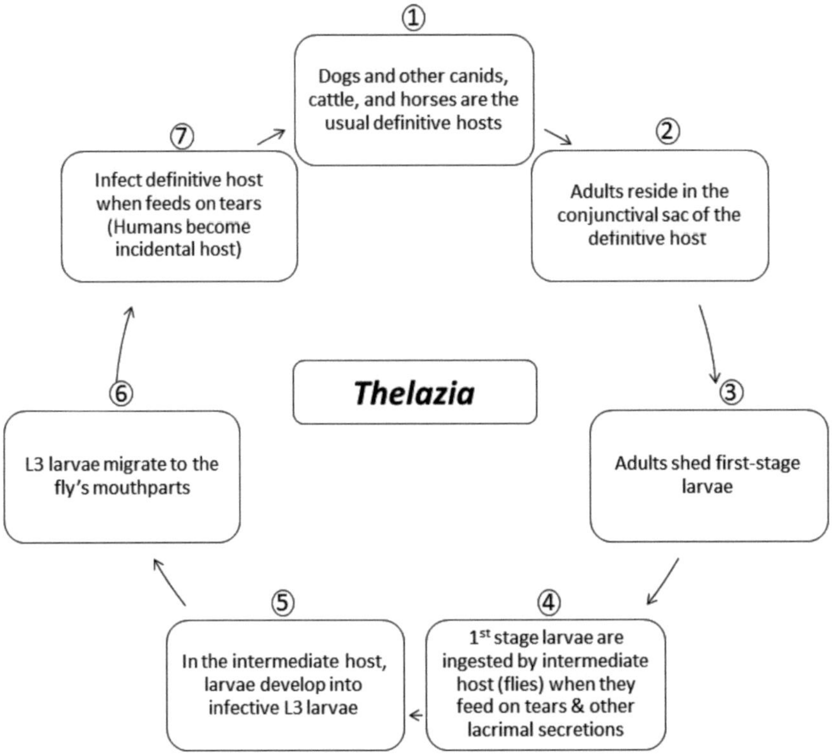

Figure 15. Life cycle of *Thelazia* (Diagrammatic representation).

5.6. Toxocariasis

Toxocariasis is caused by *Toxocara* species. *Toxocara canis* and *T. cati* are the most common species causing toxocariasis in humans worldwide, particularly in Asia, Japan, Korea, Ireland and Alabama [195–199] (Table 1, Figure 11). The life cycle of *Toxocara* involves dogs (*T. canis*)/ cats (*T. cati*) as definitive host (dog/cat). Infection is transmitted by consumption of eggs of *Toxocara* parasites, passed in the feces of definitive host (dog/cat) as shown in Figure 16. After the ingestion of eggs, larvae hatch out from the eggs in the small intestine and penetrate mucosa to migrate to different organs such as liver, lung and trachea, leading to visceral larva migrans (VLM). Sometimes, target larvae may migrate to eyes causing ocular larva migrans (OLM) [200, 201]. Host immune response is weaker in ocular larva migrans than visceral larva migrans. Various ocular clinical manifestations such as keratitis, hypopyon, iritis, uveitis, posterior pole granuloma, vitreous abscess and retinal detachment, strabismus, vision loss are attributed due to vitritis, cystoid macular edema and tractional retinal detachment [11, 202–204]. Based on clinical and physical examination, ocular toxocariasis is classified as chronic endophthalmitis, posterior granuloma and peripheral granuloma [205]. Approximately 25–50% of ocular toxocariasis patients present as posterior pole granuloma, due to lodging of the parasite in small perifoveal end-arteries, and approximately in 50% of ocular toxocariasis patients peripheral granuloma is present. Acute lesion appears as hazy, white mass in the peripheral fundus that may mimic the appearance of snowbank seen in patients with pars planitis.

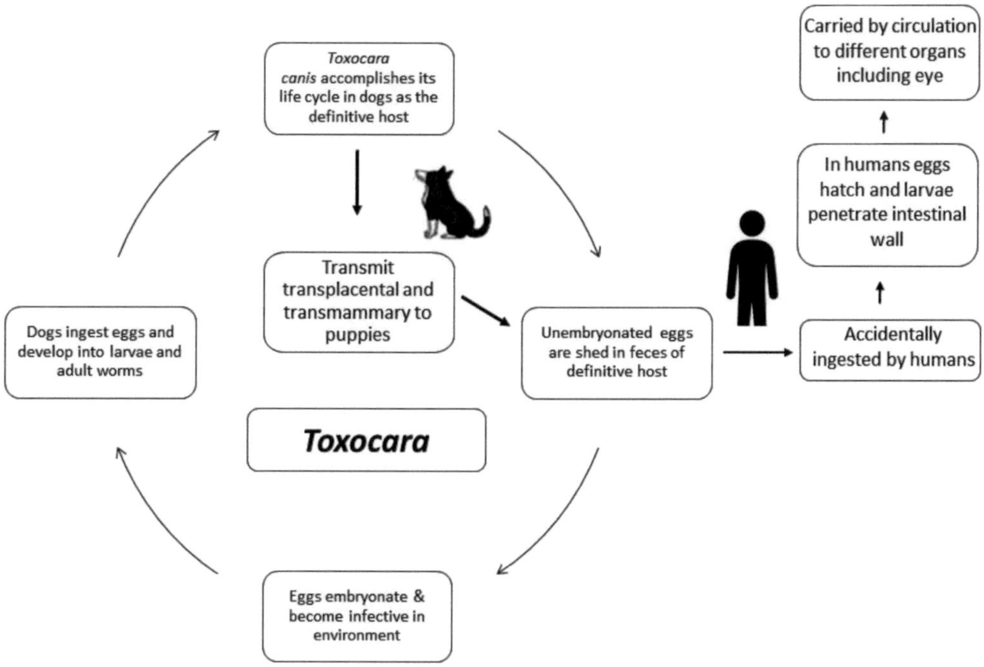

Figure 16. Life cycle of *Toxocara* (Diagrammatic representation).

High index of suspicion is required for establishing the diagnosis of OLM during ocular examination [205]. Marked eosinophilia along with positive serology by ELISA [206] helps in confirming the diagnosis [207]. Detection of specific antibodies in the vitreous fluid also helps in differentiating it from retinoblastoma [208]. ELISA based on the excretory-secretory antigens of *T. canis* reported to have a sensitivity of 78% [209]. ELISA developed by Seoul National University, using crude antigen of *Toxocara* larvae, showed a sensitivity of 92.2% and specificity of 86.6% [210]. PCR available in research laboratories [211] may help in the diagnosis of ocular toxocariasis. Nucleotide homology of 97–99% has been reported between Vietnamese *Toxocara canis* and other *Toxocara* geographical strains by comparing the nucleotide sequence of internal transcribed spacer 2 (ITS2) of ribosomal DNA of *T. canis* [212]. Although PCR has been shown to be the best diagnostic modality in animal models of ocular toxocariasis, molecular techniques are not available in hospitals of resource limiting countries [213]. Vision loss, eye inflammation or damage to the retina occurs if not treated. Prognosis is good with medical and surgical treatment [200].

Albendazole and mebendazole are the drugs of choices for the treatment of VLM [214, 215]. However, there is a limited role of antiparasitic drugs in the treatment of OLM. Photocoagulation along with steroids has been recommended for the treatment of OLM.

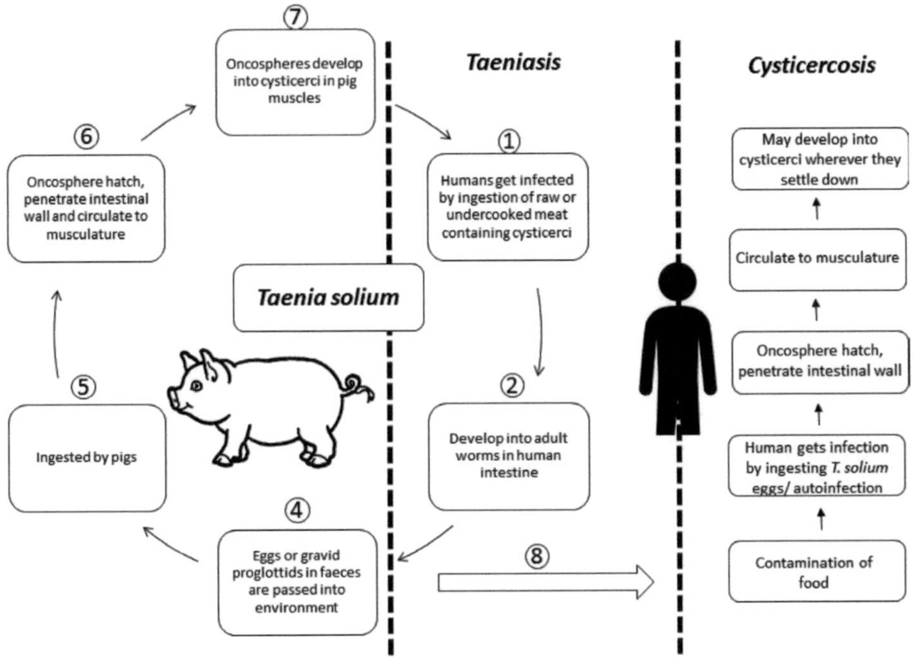

Figure 17. Life cycle of *Taenia solium* (Diagrammatic representation).

6. Cestodes infections

6.1. Cysticercosis

Cysticercosis is caused by the larval cysts of the tapeworm *Taenia solium.* Humans acquire cysticercosis infection by the consumption of food contaminated with the *Taenia solium* eggs, passed in feces of the infected humans, harboring the adult worms in their intestine as depicted in Figure 17 [216]. Autoinfection has also been reported in persons suffering from taeniasis that may result in cysticercosis. Eating of raw or uncooked pork results in adult worm infection, the taeniasis. It is considered as one of the important neglected parasitic infections (NPIs), prevalent in Asia, Africa and Latin America where poor sanitation conditions prevail (Figure 11) [217]. These larval cyst may lodge into different organs/tissues (brain, muscles, eyes or other tissues) [218], resulting in varying clinical symptoms.

Ocular involvement is well documented and several case reports have documented the orbital, intraocular, subretinal and optic nerve involvement due to cysticercosis [219, 220]. Free-floating cyst can be found in vitreous or anterior chamber of the eye. Cranial nerve or intra-ocular muscles lesions may result in gaze palsies [221–223].

Diagnosis is usually established by ophthalmoscopic examination along with imaging evidence of ultrasonography, CT scan or MRI scan. Although serology is easy to perform, it is usually negative in isolated ocular cysticercosis patient [224]. Molecular techniques such as

http://dx.doi.org/10.5772/64137

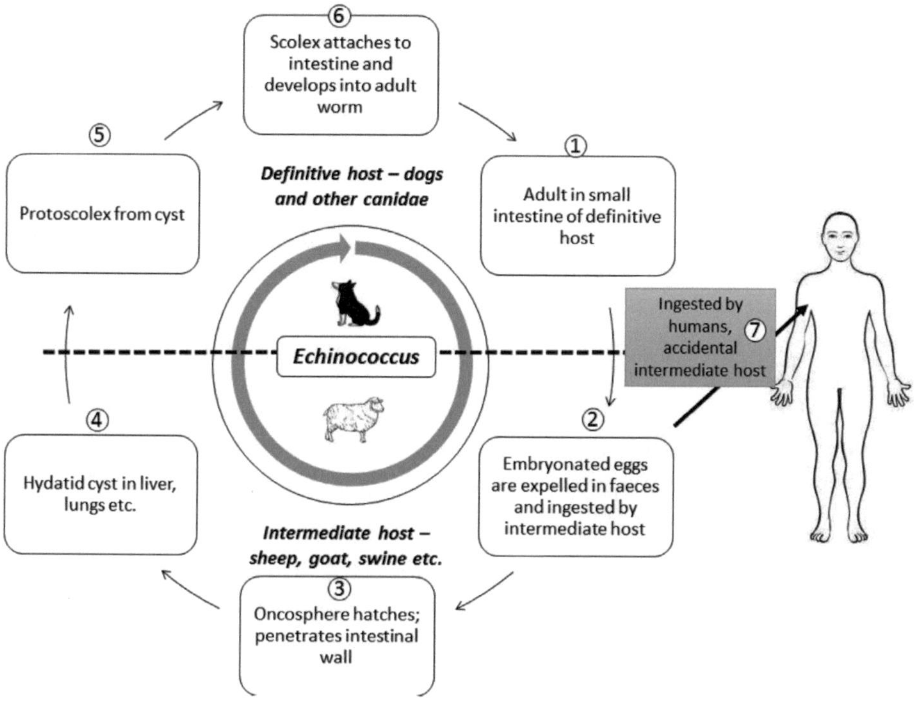

Figure 18. Life cycle of *Echinococcus* (Diagrammatic representation).

conventional PCR, real-time PCR [218] and loop-mediated isothermal amplification (LAMP) [225] can be utilized for establishing the diagnosis of ocular cysticercosis and for genotyping [30, 226]. However, it requires a sophisticated molecular laboratory setup, which is not available widely in developing nations.

Without treatment, symptoms related to visual disturbances persist. Symptoms resolve with surgical and medical treatment [227]. Albendazole along with steroids are the main drugs used in the treatment. Steroid treatment decreases the inflammatory response associated with the antihelminthic therapy around the lesions. Surgical removal of large cysts is recommended where there is an impairment of the vision [224].

6.2. Echinococcosis

Echinococcosis/hydatidosis is caused by infection of the larval stages of the *Echinococcus* spp [228], and ocular manifestations occur approximately in 1% of the cases suffering from hydatid disease [229]. Echinococcosis is mainly found in Asia, Africa, Latin America, Russia, Australia and the Mediterranean regions (Figure 11) [230]. It is acquired by the consumption of contaminated food and water with fecal matter containing eggs of *Echinococcus* parasites. The life cycle includes development of adult worms in small bowel of definitive hosts such as dogs and other canids. Eggs are passed in feces and contaminate environment as shown in Figure 18.

The symptoms and signs depend on the location of the cyst in the target organ. Most common ocular finding is the development of proptosis due to the presence of intraorbital space occupying lesion. This may further lead to exposure to keratitis and ulceration of the cornea. Other complications due to the local invasion of the expanding cyst may lead to erosion of orbital wall, optic atrophy and optic neuritis. Subretinal hydatid cyst has been reported. In severe cases, blindness may also occur [231].

The diagnosis depends on the clinical findings suggestive of hydatid cyst on ocular examination and confirmed by radiological techniques such as ultrasonography, CT scan and/or MRI [232, 233]. "Double wall" sign is a characteristic of orbital hydatid cyst seen by ultrasonography [232]. Serology may also aid in diagnosis. However, in majority of the commercially and in-house serological assays, hydatid fluid is the main antigenic component and sensitivity of IgG-ELISA reported in various studies varies from 64.8 to 100%, while specificity varies from 87.5 to 100%. Purified and recombinant antigens are also being tried for developing ELISA with high sensitivity and specificity [234]. Fine needle aspiration cytology can also be performed for establishing the diagnosis [235].

Symptoms persist if not treated [236]. Surgical removal of the cyst is the treatment of choice. Medical therapy includes administration of albendazole or mebendazole to prevent the recurrences due to the contents of the cyst leaking into the surgical sites [237]. If the cyst is accidently ruptured, in situ irrigation with hypertonic saline should be performed. However, it causes local inflammatory reaction that may lead to atrophy of optic nerve [238].

7. Trematodes infections

7.1. Fascioliasis

Fascioliasis is a food-borne parasitic infection caused by trematodes that mainly affect liver. It is acquired by eating metacercaria of *Fasciola hepatica* encysted on leaves that are eaten raw. Two important species are *Fasciola hepatica* and *F. gigantica*. The life cycle includes release of eggs from adult flukes that further develop into miracidia, sporocysts, rediae, cercariae and metacercariae as shown in Figure 19. The parasite passes its life cycle in two different hosts: sheep, goat, cattle and man act as definitive host and snails of the genus *Lymnaea* act as intermediate host. The eggs are passed out in the feces of definitive hosts that mature in water. Ciliated miracidium develops inside each egg in 2–3 weeks. Miracidium after getting released from egg finds its way to its suitable intermediate host. Inside the lymph spaces of the molluscan host, the miracidium passes through stages of sporocyst, two generations of rediae and finally to the stage of cercariae. The mature cercariae escape from the snail into the water and encyst (metacercariae) in blades of grass or water-cress, which is ingested by herbivorous animals and occasionally by man. On entering the digestive tract, the metacercariae excyst in the duodenum and migrate through intestinal wall into peritoneal cavity. It further traverses through liver capsule, parenchyma and ultimately settle in the biliary passages, where it mature into adults. The eggs are liberated in the feces through bile, completing the life cycle.

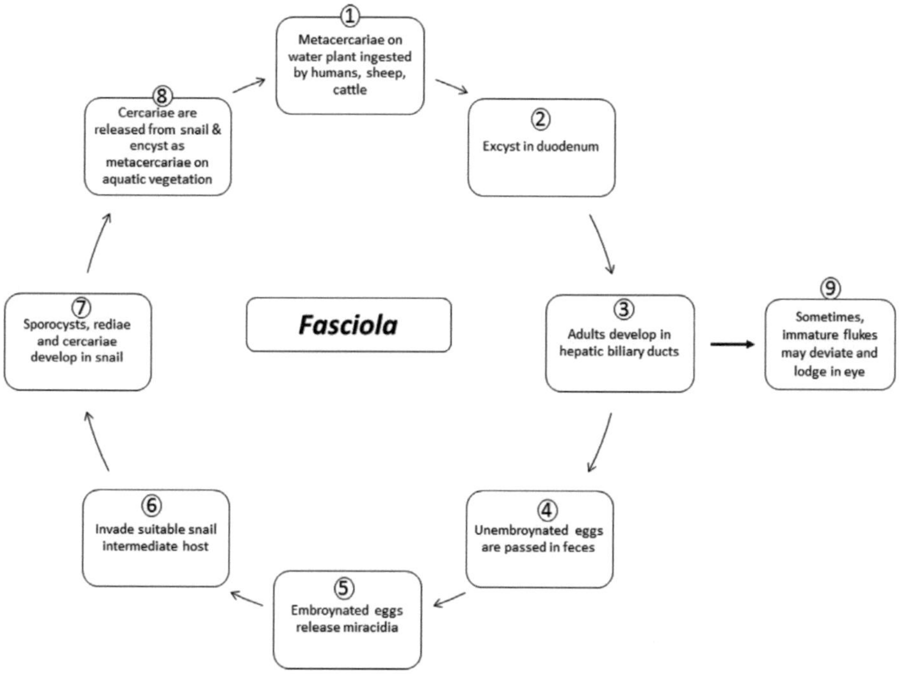

Figure 19. Life cycle of *Fasciola* (Diagrammatic representation).

Opthalmofascioliasis is the term used for those cases in which eye infection is directly caused by migrant ectopic fasciolid fluke. All other patients with ocular manifestations due to fasciolids located in liver or other organs should be classified as fascioliasis with ocular implications. Although ocular involvement in fascioliasis is rare, cases have been reported from France, Spain, Italy, Austria, Belgium, United Kingdom, Algeria, Tunisia, Iran, Uzbekistan, Korea, China, Argentina, Chile, Peru, Brazil and Guatemala (Figure 20) [239]. Symptoms and signs usually relate to the affected eye and may cause conjunctival hyperaemia, corneal oedema, dilated episcleral vessels, paralysis of extraocular muscles, decrease in perception of light, deep anterior chamber with flare, uveitis and so on. Diagnosis is established directly by visualization of leaf-shaped like organism in the eye or by studying the morphological features of the surgically removed worm. Eosinophilia, positive serology by ELISA or presence of eggs in stools may aid in diagnosis. Severe complications may occur if not treated. Early surgical intervention is associated with rapid response and reasonable final visual acuity [14]. Thus, ophthalmological manifestations have been known to be cured with surgical treatment without any antiparasitic treatment [14]. However, triclabendazole is the drug of choice if medical treatment is required.

7.2. Schistosomiasis

Schistosomiasis, or bilharziasis, is caused by trematode flatworm of the genus *Schistosoma*. Freshwater snails release the larval forms in the water, which penetrate the skin of human host

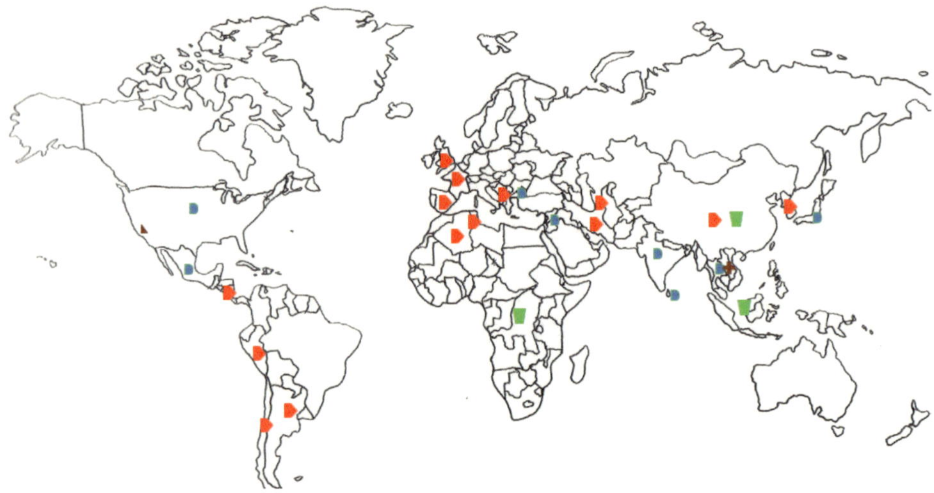

Figure 20. World map showing geographical areas endemic for ocular trematode infections.

while swimming, bathing, fishing and even domestic chores such as laundry and herding livestock. In the human body, the larvae mature into adult schistosomes, which reside in the blood vessels. Eggs released by females are passed out of the body in the urine or feces. It is prevalent in sub-Saharan Africa, China and South Asia (Figure 20) [8].

Ocular involvement is not the usual site that is involved in schistosomiasis, but cases have been reported where Schistosoma ova or even the adult worm can reach the systemic circulation and can lodge itself at ectopic sites such as eyes. Although schistosomiasis is very common, ocular cases are rare. It can cause uveitis or subretinal granuloma [240]. Diagnosis is established by direct demonstration of eggs/cercariae in the eye. Detection of eggs in the urine and feces may aid in establishing the diagnosis. Symptoms persist if not treated. Praziquantel is the drug of choice for all forms of schistosomiasis [8].

7.3. Other rare ocular infections by trematodes

The cases of acute nodular conjunctivitis and anterior chamber granuloma formation have been documented, which are caused by endemic water-borne trematode infection. The identification of the remnants of parasites aspirated from such cases revealed that these parasites belong to the genus *Philophthalmus* that are known to parasitize birds [25, 241]. Humans acquire infection accidently while bathing or playing in contaminated water. Conjunctival nodules heal spontaneously, and anterior chamber nodules can be treated with topical/oral corticosteroids. Surgical removal is recommended in cases having large nodules. First human case of *Clinostomum* lacramalitis was reported in Thailand [242]. Human cases of intraocular infection with mesocercariae of *Alaria americana* and other *Alaria* mesocercariae have been reported in patients who had ingested undercooked contaminated frogs legs [243].

http://dx.doi.org/10.5772/64137

8. Eye infections caused by ectoparasites

8.1. Myiasis

Myiasis is an infection caused by larvae of flies. It is common in tropical and subtropical areas. It is known as ophthalmomyiasis when ocular structures are involved. Ophthalmomyiasis is categorized into three clinical categories (ophthalmomyiasis externa, ophthalmomyiasis interna and orbital myiasis), depending on the location of larvae in the eyes. Several genera have been reported to cause myiasis such as *Dermatobia, Gasterophilus, Oestra, Cordylobia, Chrysomyia, Wohlfahrtia, Cochliomyia* and *Hypoderma* [1]. Significantly, larvae causing ophthalmomyiasis belong to the genus *Hypoderma* [16]. *Three cases of external* ophthalmomyiasis, two due to *Oestrus ovis and one due to Cochliomyia hominivorax* were reported earlier from North India [17]. *Oestra ovis* also known as sheep nasal botfly is responsible for causing ophthalmomyiasis externa in shepherding areas [244–247]. It mainly involves eyelids, conjunctiva, lacrimal sac and nasolacrimal ducts. Most common clinical feature is the foreign body sensation and may be associated with conjunctivitis and keratitis.

Diagnosis is established by the identification of the maggots. Treatment usually involves the surgical removal of the maggots. Medical treatment involves just one oral dose (150 to 200 μg/kg of body weight) of ivermectin [16]. However, the use of ivermectin for the treatment of myiasis is an off-label treatment in many countries and should be used for selected cases. The side effects such as dermal eruptions, fever, dizziness, migraines and muscular pains are common. Antibiotics and steroids may also be required to prevent the inflammation and superadded bacterial infection. Opthalmomyiasis interna [248] is caused by the invasion of the ocular structures leading to uveitis, lens dislocation and retinal detachment. Diagnosis is established by visualizing the migratory tracks along subretina by the ophthalmoscopy. Symptoms persist if not treated. Serious complications may also occur such as lens dislocation and retinal detachment due to invasion of tissue [1]. Steroid therapy is advocated if there is severe inflammation, and surgical removal is performed in severe cases. Orbital myiasis is seen in patients who are not able to maintain good personal hygiene [16]. Treatment is directed at removal of maggots and control of secondary infection. Preventive measures include maintenance of good sanitation conditions and proper disposal of waste material to control the flies in surrounding areas.

8.2. Lice

Important genera of the lice causing human infestation belong to *Pediculus* and *Phthirus.* Geographical areas where *Phthiriasis palpebrarum* is commonly found have been depicted in Table 1 and Figure 21. Eggs or nits laid down by lice glue themselves to body hairs or clothing fibers. Nymphs emerge from eggs and feed on the host, causing pruritis. Eyebrows and eyelashes are most commonly, involved. Excoriation marks along with small erythematous papules aid in diagnosis. Nits can be found at the base of eyelashes, substantiating the clinical diagnosis. Symptoms persist if not treated. Eyelid disease is treated by petrolatum and non-eyelid involvement may be treated with lindane, permethrin, pyrethrin or malathion [1].

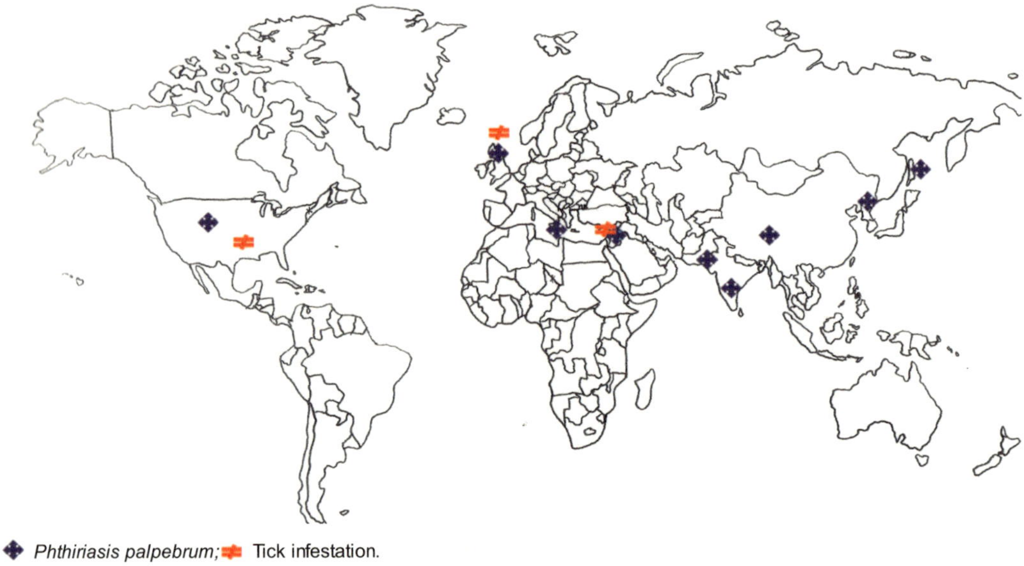

Figure 21. World map showing geographical areas endemic for ocular ectoparasites. *Phthiriasis palpebrarum*; Tick infestation.

8.3. Ticks

Ticks belonging to the class Arachnida are important vectors for the transmission of several infections to humans [1]. Geographical regions where ticks' infestation has been reported are depicted in Table 1 and Figure 21. Ticks complete their life cycle in three different stages, i.e. larva, nymph and adult, and all the life cycle stages require blood meals. Ticks have been reported to attach to ocular structures that may appear as meibomian gland mass. Symptoms persist if not treated. Treatment includes removal of ticks, and tick bite granuloma may resolve after several weeks.

9. Summary

Ocular parasitic infections are of medical importance worldwide because of significant morbidity rates, and if not diagnosed and treated on time could lead to vision loss. High index of clinical suspicion is required to establish the diagnosis for further confirmation by laboratory techniques followed by specific treatment. Direct demonstration of the parasite is possible in few ocular parasitic infections, while in few, specific clinical features such as changes in retina on direct ocular examination may point toward specific diagnosis. Serology has limited role in the diagnosis as most of the ocular parasitic infections are localized in the eye. Utility of different diagnostic techniques in various parasitic ocular infections has been summarized in Table 2. Although reports reveal that the serology for antibody detection and/or molecular techniques for parasite DNA detection, when applied directly on the ocular tissues, aqueous or vitreous humor usually confirm the diagnosis, these techniques have its own merits and demerits. IgG immunoblot technique has been applied for the diagnosis of ocular toxoplasmosis with some success, and it is suggested that local antibody production is presumed to have occurred, if immunoreactive bands are detected in the aqueous humor but not in the serum [249]. Future reports in this direction may throw further light on its utility. Moreover, application of Western blotting technique may be possible only in limited diagnostic centers.

Report on "Diagnostic Approach to Ocular Toxoplasmosis" revealed in conclusion that the clinical diagnosis of ocular toxoplasmosis may be supported by laboratory tests in 60–85% of cases, depending on the time of sampling. Analysis of the aqueous humor is particularly helpful in patients with atypical lesions or in individuals who are irresponsive to specific therapy. Even so, a laboratory confirmation of the clinical diagnosis is not achieved in 15–40% of cases [72].

In general, it can be concluded that the clinical awareness and multiple approaches/techniques for the confirmatory diagnosis of clinically suspected ocular parasitic infections may yield higher sensitivity and diagnostic efficacy, as suggested earlier [250].

Treatment depends on the causative agent and may involve surgical removal and/or medical treatment with antiparasitic drugs (Table 2). In few infections, steroids are also prescribed to prevent the damage from the inflammatory response associated with the dying parasites. Preventive strategies depend on the type of parasitic infection and mainly include control of vector population for vector borne parasitic infections, maintenance of good personal hygiene and providing awareness to people about ocular parasitic infections through information, education and communication (IEC).

The need of increased awareness and clinical suspicion of OPI for prompt and specific diagnosis followed by application of sensitive and specific diagnostic technique(s) for confirmation and effective treatment are the main challenges.

The future research priorities need to be directed to study exact host-pathogen mechanisms, local immune responses and to establish more sensitive and specific diagnostic techniques. The molecular techniques can provide rapid diagnosis of multiple ocular parasitic infections and species identification for specific therapy. Multiplex PCR assay, if developed, can add new dimensions in the diagnosis. Efforts to develop animal models are desired that may further help to study the exact host-pathogen mechanisms, local immune responses and in developing new treatment strategies.

Ocular protozoal infections	**Diagnosis**	**Treatment**
Toxoplasmosis	Serology – IgM, IgG, IgA Molecular: PCR, Real-time PCR	a. Pyrimethamine and sulfadiazine plus corticosteroids b. Trimethoprim/sulfamethoxazole plus oral prednisolone c. Intravitreal clindamycin (1-1.5mg) injection and dexamethasone d. Surgery reserved for severe complicated cases

Ocular protozoal infections	**Diagnosis**	**Treatment**
Acanthamoeba keratitis	Microscopy, culture on non-nutrient plates (coated with bacteria)/ in flasks (PBS +Bacteria), PCR, Real-time PCR	a. Biguanides – PHMB (0.02%) b. Chlorhexidine 0.02% in combination with aromatic diamidines such as 0.1% propamidine isethionate, 0.15% dibromopropamidine, hexamidine 0.1% and neomycin (Topical antimicrobials should be administered every hourly for first several days and there after frequency reduced to every 3 hours with a minimum duration of therapy of 3-4 weeks c. Surgical treatment includes keratoplasty or its variation known as DALK (Deep Anterior Lamellar Keratoplasty)
Chagas disease	Blood smear, Buffy coat, culture, xenodiagnoses and PCR	a. Benznidazole 5-10 mg/kg daily in 2-3 divided doses for 60 days b. Nifurtimox 15 mg/kg daily in 3 divided doses for 60-90 days
Malaria	Thin and thick blood film for microscopy, antigen detection, PCR	a. *Plasmodium vivax* – Chloroquine + primaquine b. *P. falciparum* – Artemisinin combination therapy (Artemisinin + sulfadoxine-pyrimethamine or artemisinin + lumefantrine) as per WHO guidelines
Leishmaniasis	Microscopy of tissue smears, culture on NNN media, PCR	Pentavalent antimonial compounds, liposomal amphotericin B, miltefosine (dose is weight dependent), paromomycin, azoles such as ketoconazole, itraconazole and fluconazole
Microsporidiosis	Microscopy, Immunofluorescence assay, PCR	Topical fumagillin bicylohexylammonium (Fumidil B) 3 mg/mL in saline (fumagillin 70 μg/mL) eye drops: two drops every 2 hours for 4 days, then two drops four times daily (investigational use only in United States) plus albendazole 400 mg orally twice daily for management of systemic infection.
Giardiasis	Confirming by intestinal infection	Metronidazole, tinidazole, and nitazoxanide. Others include paromomycin, quinacrine, and furazolidone
Ocular nematode infections		
Onchocerciasis	Slit-lamp examination, Biopsy of skin to identify larvae, skin nodules examination for identification of adult worms, PCR, antibody detection	a. Ivermectin: given every 6 months for the life span of the adult worm or as long as infected person has evidence of skin or eye infection b. New treatment: Doxycycline, before starting treatment infection with *Loa loa* has to be ruled out c. Removal of adult worms

http://dx.doi.org/10.5772/64137

Ocular protozoal infections	**Diagnosis**	**Treatment**
Loiasis		a. Surgical removal of the worm under the skin or across the eye b. Diethylcarbamazine (DEC) is the drug of choice c. Albendazole is given to patients not responding to DEC
Dirofilariasis		a. Surgical removal of the worm b. DEC is given for medical treatment
Gnathostomiasis	Identification of the removed worm Serology to detect antibodies	a. Surgical removal of worm
Thelaziasis	b. Identification of worm removed from conjunctival sac c. Eggs and larvae may be seen by microscopy of tears and other eye secretions	Removal of worm
Toxocariasis	Histological demonstration of toxocara larva Serology by ELISA	d. Topical and systemic corticosteroids are useful in managing intraocular inflammation e. Role of anthelmintic therapy in ocular toxocariasis remains unclear f. Recommended drugs for systemic toxocariasis are: g. Albendazole 400mg given twice daily for 7-14 days h. Diethylcarbamazine - given at 3-4 mg/kg/day for 21 days
Ocular cestode infections		
Cysticercosis	Imaging with MRI, CT scan and USG Serology	a. Antiparasitic drugs – Albendazole 15mg/kg/day for 4 weeks, Praziquantel b. Corticosteroids in tapering dose over a period of 1 month c. Surgery
Echinococcosis	Imaging	a. Surgical removal b. Albendazole is given as an anti-infective prophylaxis
Ocular trematode infections		
Fascioliasis	Detection of adult worm in the eye Other features such as eosinophilia, stool examination and serology may help	a. Surgical removal of worm b. Triclabendazole 10mg/kg body weight as a single dose

Ocular protozoal infections	Diagnosis	Treatment
Schistosomiasis	Stool and urine examination for detection of parasitic eggs or detection of eggs or cercariae in eye Serology	Praziquantel 40-60mg/kg per day in two to three divided doses for one day
Philopthalmosis	Identification of the remnants of parasites aspirated from such cases	a. Conjunctival nodules heal spontaneously and anterior chamber nodules can be treated with topical/ oral corticosteroids. b. Surgical removal is recommended in cases having large nodules
Ocular infections by ectoparasites		
Myiasis	a. Identification of the maggots b. Visualizing the migratory tracks along sub retina	a. Surgical removal of the maggots b. Ivermectin 150-200 μg/kg of body weight in single dose c. Steroid therapy
Phthiriasis palpebrum	a. Excoriation marks along with small erythematous papules b. Nits can be found at the base of eyelashes	a. Eyelid disease is treated by petrolatum b. Non-eyelid involvement may be treated with lindane, permethrin, pyrethin or malathion
Tick infestation	Biomicroscopy may reveal ticks	Removal of ticks

Table 2. Diagnosis and treatment of various ocular parasitic infections

Author details

Nancy Malla* and Kapil Goyal

*Address all correspondence to: drmallanancy@gmail.com

Department of Medical Parasitology, Postgraduate Institute of Medical Education and Research, Chandigarh, India

References

[1] Klotz SA, Penn CC, Negvesky GJ, Butrus SI. Fungal and parasitic infections of the eye. Clinical microbiology reviews. 2000;13(4):662-85.

[2] Chawla A, Armstrong M, Carley F. Acanthamoeba keratitis – an increasing incidence. Contact lens & anterior eye : the journal of the British Contact Lens Association. 2014;37(2):120.

[3] Lorenzo-Morales J, Martin-Navarro CM, Lopez-Arencibia A, Arnalich-Montiel F, Pinero JE, Valladares B. Acanthamoeba keratitis: an emerging disease gathering importance worldwide? Trends in parasitology. 2013;29(4):181-7.

[4] Montoya JG, Liesenfeld O. Toxoplasmosis. Lancet. 2004;363(9425):1965-76.

[5] Sharma S, Pasricha G, Das D, Aggarwal RK. Acanthamoeba keratitis in non-contact lens wearers in India: DNA typing-based validation and a simple detection assay. Archives of ophthalmology. 2004;122(10):1430-4.

[6] Gopinathan U, Sharma S, Garg P, Rao GN. Review of epidemiological features, microbiological diagnosis and treatment outcome of microbial keratitis: experience of over a decade. Indian journal of ophthalmology. 2009;57(4):273-9.

[7] Sharma S, Garg P, Rao GN. Patient characteristics, diagnosis, and treatment of non-contact lens related Acanthamoeba keratitis. The British journal of ophthalmology. 2000;84(10):1103-8.

[8] Nimir AR, Saliem A, Ibrahim IA. Ophthalmic parasitosis: a review article. Interdisciplinary Perspectives on Infectious Diseases. 2012;2012:587402.

[9] Joseph J, Vemuganti GK, Sharma S. Microsporidia: emerging ocular pathogens. Indian journal of medical microbiology. 2005;23(2):80-91.

[10] Malla N, Aggarwal AK, Mahajan RC. A serological study of human toxocariasis in north India. The National medical journal of India. 2002;15(3):145-7.

[11] Fomda BA, Ahmad Z, Khan NN, Tanveer S, Wani SA. Ocular toxocariasis in a child: a case report from Kashmir, north India. Indian journal of medical microbiology. 2007;25(4):411-2.

[12] Prabhakar SK, Vijaykumar GS, Mahesh BS, Shanthamallappa. Human ocular thelaziasis: a case report from Karnataka. Indian journal of medical microbiology. 2015;33(2):324-5.

[13] Sachdeva RS, Manchanda SK, Abrol S, Wadhwa SC, Ramachandran KA. Freely mobile cysticercus in the anterior chamber. Indian journal of ophthalmology. 1995;43(3):135-6.

[14] Dalimi A, Jabarvand M. Fasciola hepatica in the human eye. Transactions of the Royal Society of Tropical Medicine and Hygiene. 2005;99(10):798-800.

[15] Joshi G, Parchand S, Dogra MR, Gupta PK, Khurana S, Gupta V, et al. Live juvenile strobilate tapeworm in the anterior chamber of the human eye. Archives of ophthalmology. 2012;130(11):1464-6.

[16] Francesconi F, Lupi O. Myiasis. Clinical microbiology reviews. 2012;25(1):79-105.

[17] Khurana S, Biswal M, Bhatti HS, Pandav SS, Gupta A, Chatterjee SS, et al. Ophthalmomyiasis: three cases from North India. Indian journal of medical microbiology. 2010;28(3):257-61.

[18] Sulyok M, Rozsa L, Bodo I, Tappe D, Hardi R. Ocular pentastomiasis in the Democratic Republic of the Congo. PLoS neglected tropical diseases. 2014;8(7):e3041.

[19] Tan SY, Liu SW, Jiang SB. HIV/AIDS and ocular complications. International Journal of Ophthalmology. 2009;2(2):95-105.

[20] Couture S, Agrawal R, Woods K, Lockwood D, Pavesio CE, Addison PKF. A case of panuveitis with hypopyon due to presumed ocular leishmaniasis in a HIV patient. Journal of Opthalmic Inflammation and Infection. 2014;4(21):1-5.

[21] Bacon AS, Dart JK, Ficker LA, Matheson MM, Wright P. Acanthamoeba keratitis. The value of early diagnosis. Ophthalmology. 1993;100(8):1238-43.

[22] Lalitha P, Lin CC, Srinivasan M, Mascarenhas J, Prajna NV, Keenan JD, et al. Acanthamoeba keratitis in South India: a longitudinal analysis of epidemics. Ophthalmic Epidemiology. 2012;19(2):111-5.

[23] Lowder CY. Ocular microsporidiosis. International ophthalmology clinics. 1993;33(1):145-51.

[24] Lim SJ, Lee SE, Kim SH, Hong SH, You YS, Kwon OW, et al. Prevalence of Toxoplasma gondii and Toxocara canis among patients with uveitis. Ocular immunology and inflammation. 2014;22(5):360-6.

[25] Otranto D, Eberhard ML. Zoonotic helminths affecting the human eye. Parasites & vectors. 2011;4:41.

[26] Hirst LW. Ocular infections – diagnosis. Australian family physician. 1991;20(2): 133-4, 7-45, 49.

[27] Rao NA. A laboratory approach to rapid diagnosis of ocular infections and prospects for the future. American journal of ophthalmology. 1989;107(3):283-91.

[28] Khurana S, Singh G, Bhatti HS, Malla N. Human subcutaneous dirofilariasis in India: a report of three cases with brief review of literature. Indian journal of medical microbiology. 2010;28(4):394-6.

[29] Cortez RT, Ramirez G, Collet L, Giuliari GP. Ocular parasitic diseases: a review on toxocariasis and diffuse unilateral subacute neuroretinitis. Journal of pediatric ophthalmology and strabismus. 2011;48(4):204-12.

[30] Sharma M, Beke N, Khurana S, Bhatti HS, Sehgal R, Malla N. An Ocular cysticercosis case: caused by Asian Genotype of Taenia solium. Indian journal of Medical Microbiology. 2015;33(4)583-585.

[31] Hogan RN, Jakobiec FA. Molecular pathological diagnosis of ocular infections. International ophthalmology clinics. 1996;36(3):223-46.

[32] Rathinam SR, Annamalai R, Biswas J. Intraocular parasitic infections. Ocular immunology and inflammation. 2011;19(5):327-36.

[33] Pasricha G, Sharma S, Garg P, Aggarwal RK. Use of 18S rRNA gene-based PCR assay for diagnosis of acanthamoeba keratitis in non-contact lens wearers in India. Journal of Clinical Microbiology. 2003;41(7):3206-11.

[34] Basu S, Sharma S, Kar S, Das T. DNA chip-assisted diagnosis of a previously unknown etiology of intermediate uveitis – Toxoplasma gondii. Indian journal of ophthalmology. 2010;58(6):535-7.

[35] Sharma S. Diagnosis of infectious diseases of the eye. Eye. 2012;26(2):177-84.

[36] Rathinam SR, Arya LK, Usha KR, Prajna L, Tandon V. Novel etiological agent: molecular evidence for trematode-induced anterior uveitis in children. Archives of ophthalmology. 2012;130(11):1481-4.

[37] Nath R, Gogoi R, Bordoloi N, Gogoi T. Ocular dirofilariasis. Indian journal of Pathology & Microbiology. 2010;53(1):157-9.

[38] Pushker N, Bajaj MS, Chandra M, Neena. Ocular and orbital cysticercosis. Acta ophthalmologica Scandinavica. 2001;79(4):408-13.

[39] Gomez Morales A, Croxatto JO, Crovetto L, Ebner R. Hydatid cysts of the orbit. A review of 35 cases. Ophthalmology. 1988;95(8):1027-32.

[40] Malla N, Goyal M, Pillai P, Ganguly NK, Mahajan RC. Experimental ocular toxoplasmosis with RH strain of Toxoplasma gondii. Japanese journal of experimental medicine. 1988;58(6):279-81.

[41] Takayanagi TH, Akao N, Suzuki R, Tomoda M, Tsukidate S, Fujita K. New animal model for human ocular toxocariasis: ophthalmoscopic observation. The British journal of ophthalmology. 1999;83(8):967-72.

[42] Malhotra A, Minja FJ, Crum A, Burrowes D. Ocular anatomy and cross-sectional imaging of the eye. Semin Ultrasound CT MR. 2011;32(1):2-13.

[43] Kaplan HJ. Anatomy and function of the eye. Chemical Immunology and Allergy. 2007;92:4-10.

[44] Paalman MH. Anatomy in the eye. Anatomical Record. 2000;261(6):221.

[45] Kolb H. Gross Anatomy of the Eye. 2005 May 1 [Updated 2007 May 1]. In: Kolb H, Fernandez E, Nelson R, editors. Webvision: The Organization of the Retina and Visual System [Internet]. Salt Lake City (UT): University of Utah Health Sciences Center; 1995. Available from: http://www.ncbi.nlm.nih.gov/books/NBK11534/

[46] Iveson-Iveson J. Anatomy and physiology: the eye. Nursing Mirror. 1979;148(8):31-3.

[47] Shitole S, Jakkal T, Khaire B. Inverse Bell's phenomenon: rare ophthalmic finding following ptosis surgery. Journal of clinical and diagnostic research: JCDR. 2015;9(3):ND01-2.

[48] Kageyama M, Nakatsuka K, Yamaguchi T, Owen RL, Shimada T. Ocular defense mechanisms with special reference to the demonstration and functional morphology of the conjunctiva-associated lymphoid tissue in Japanese monkeys. Archives of Histology and Cytology. 2006;69(5):311-22.

[49] Lerman S. Free radical damage and defense mechanisms in the ocular lens. Lens and eye toxicity research. 1992;9(1):9-24.

[50] Bito LZ. Species differences in the responses of the eye to irritation and trauma: a hypothesis of divergence in ocular defense mechanisms, and the choice of experimental animals for eye research. Experimental Eye Research. 1984;39(6):807-29.

[51] Chandler JW, Gillette TE. Immunologic defense mechanisms of the ocular surface. Ophthalmology. 1983;90(6):585-91.

[52] Lemp MA, Blackman HJ. Ocular surface defense mechanisms. Annals of ophthalmology. 1981;13(1):61-3.

[53] McDermott AM. Defensins and other antimicrobial peptides at the ocular surface. The ocular surface. 2004;2(4):229-47.

[54] Cunningham ET, Jr., Belfort R, Jr., Muccioli C, Arevalo JF, Zierhut M. Ocular toxoplasmosis. Ocular immunology and inflammation. 2015;23(3):191-3.

[55] Kijlstra A, Petersen E. Epidemiology, pathophysiology, and the future of ocular toxoplasmosis. Ocular immunology and inflammation. 2014;22(2):138-47.

[56] Robert-Gangneux F, Darde ML. Epidemiology of and diagnostic strategies for toxoplasmosis. Clinical microbiology reviews. 2012;25(2):264-96.

[57] Petersen E, Kijlstra A, Stanford M. Epidemiology of ocular toxoplasmosis. Ocular immunology and inflammation. 2012;20(2):68-75.

[58] Ho-Yen DO. Epidemiology of toxoplasmosis. Archives of pediatrics. 2003;10(Suppl 1): 3-4.

[59] Lachenmaier SM, Deli MA, Meissner M, Liesenfeld O. Intracellular transport of Toxoplasma gondii through the blood-brain barrier. Journal of neuroimmunology. 2011;232(1-2):119-30.

[60] Peixoto-Rangel AL, Miller EN, Castellucci L, Jamieson SE, Peixe RG, Elias Lde S, et al. Candidate gene analysis of ocular toxoplasmosis in Brazil: evidence for a role for toll-like receptor 9 (TLR9). Memorias do Instituto Oswaldo Cruz. 2009;104(8):1187-90.

[61] Pleyer U, Schluter D, Manz M. Ocular toxoplasmosis: recent aspects of pathophysiology and clinical implications. Ophthalmic Research. 2014;52(3):116-23.

[62] Holland GN. Ocular toxoplasmosis: a global reassessment. Part II: disease manifestations and management. American journal of ophthalmology. 2004;137(1):1-17.

[63] O'Connor GR. Manifestations and management of ocular toxoplasmosis. Bulletin of the New York Academy of Medicine. 1974;50(2):192-210.

[64] Park YH, Nam HW. Clinical features and treatment of ocular toxoplasmosis. The Korean journal of parasitology. 2013;51(4):393-9.

[65] Harper TW, Miller D, Schiffman JC, Davis JL. Polymerase chain reaction analysis of aqueous and vitreous specimens in the diagnosis of posterior segment infectious uveitis. American journal of ophthalmology. 2009;147(1):140-7 e2.

[66] Cassaing S, Bessieres MH, Berry A, Berrebi A, Fabre R, Magnaval JF. Comparison between two amplification sets for molecular diagnosis of toxoplasmosis by real-time PCR. Journal of Clinical Microbiology. 2006;44(3):720-4.

[67] Robert-Gangneux F, Sterkers Y, Yera H, Accoceberry I, Menotti J, Cassaing S, et al. Molecular diagnosis of toxoplasmosis in immunocompromised patients: a 3-year multicenter retrospective study. Journal of Clinical Microbiology. 2015;53(5):1677-84.

[68] Filisetti D, Sterkers Y, Brenier-Pinchart MP, Cassaing S, Dalle F, Delhaes L, et al. Multicentric comparative assessment of the bio-evolution Toxoplasma gondii detection kit with eight laboratory-developed PCR assays for molecular diagnosis of congenital toxoplasmosis. Journal of Clinical Microbiology. 2015;53(1):29-34.

[69] Hashoosh DA, Majeed IA. Comparison of two assays in the diagnosis of toxoplasmosis: immunological and molecular. Eastern Mediterranean Health Journal. 2014;20(1): 46-50.

[70] Remington JS, Thulliez P, Montoya JG. Recent developments for diagnosis of toxoplasmosis. Journal of Clinical Microbiology. 2004;42(3):941-5.

[71] Bou G, Figueroa MS, Marti-Belda P, Navas E, Guerrero A. Value of PCR for detection of Toxoplasma gondii in aqueous humor and blood samples from immunocompetent patients with ocular toxoplasmosis. Journal of Clinical Microbiology. 1999;37(11): 3465-8.

[72] Garweg JG, de Groot-Mijnes JD, Montoya JG. Diagnostic approach to ocular toxoplasmosis. Ocular Immunology and Inflammation. 2011;19(4):255-61.

[73] Khurana S, Bagga R, Aggarwal A, Lyngdoh V, Shivapriya, Diddi K, et al. Serological screening for antenatal toxoplasma infection in India. Indian Journal of Medical Microbiology. 2010;28(2):143-6.

[74] Singh MP, Dubey ML, Sud A, Malla N. Antibody response to Toxoplasma gondii in saliva samples from human immunodeficiency virus-infected patients. British Journal of Biomedical Science. 2005;62(2):81-4.

[75] Zargar AH, Masoodi SR, Laway BA, Sofi BA, Wani AI. Seroprevalence of toxoplasmosis in women with repeated abortions in Kashmir. Journal of Epidemiology & Community Health. 1998;52(2):135-6.

[76] Thokar MA, Malla N, Wattal C. Serological study of patients clinically suspected to have toxoplasmosis in Kashmir. Indian Journal of Medical Research. 1988;88:29-34.

[77] Delair E, Monnet D, Grabar S, Dupouy-Camet J, Yera H, Brezin AP. Respective roles of acquired and congenital infections in presumed ocular toxoplasmosis. American Journal of Ophthalmology. 2008;146(6):851-5.

[78] de Boer JH, Luyendijk L, Rothova A, Kijlstra A. Analysis of ocular fluids for local antibody production in uveitis. The British Journal of Ophthalmology. 1995;79(6):610-6.

[79] Garweg JG, Jacquier P, Boehnke M. Early aqueous humor analysis in patients with human ocular toxoplasmosis. Journal of Clinical Microbiology. 2000;38(3):996-1001.

[80] Lima GS, Saraiva PG, Saraiva FP. Current therapy of acquired ocular toxoplasmosis: a review. Journal of Ocular Pharmacology and Therapeutics : The Official Journal of the Association for Ocular Pharmacology and Therapeutics. 2015;31(9):511-7.

[81] Holland GN, Lewis KG. An update on current practices in the management of ocular toxoplasmosis. American Journal of Ophthalmology. 2002;134(1):102-14.

[82] Siddiqui R, Khan NA. Biology and pathogenesis of Acanthamoeba. Parasites & Vectors. 2012;5:6.

[83] Bharathi JM, Srinivasan M, Ramakrishnan R, Meenakshi R, Padmavathy S, Lalitha PN. A study of the spectrum of Acanthamoeba keratitis: a three-year study at a tertiary eye care referral center in South India. Indian Journal of Ophthalmology. 2007;55(1):37-42.

[84] Vaddavalli PK, Garg P, Sharma S, Sangwan VS, Rao GN, Thomas R. Role of confocal microscopy in the diagnosis of fungal and acanthamoeba keratitis. Ophthalmology. 2011;118(1):29-35.

[85] Winchester K, Mathers WD, Sutphin JE, Daley TE. Diagnosis of Acanthamoeba keratitis in vivo with confocal microscopy. Cornea. 1995;14(1):10-7.

[86] Goldschmidt P, Degorge S, Benallaoua D, Saint-Jean C, Batellier L, Alouch C, et al. New tool for the simultaneous detection of 10 different genotypes of Acanthamoeba available from the American Type Culture Collection. The British Journal of Ophthalmology. 2009;93(8):1096-100.

[87] Hauber S, Parkes H, Siddiqui R, Khan NA. The use of high-resolution (1)H nuclear magnetic resonance (NMR) spectroscopy in the clinical diagnosis of Acanthamoeba. Parasitology Research. 2011;109(6):1661-9.

[88] Lorenzo-Morales J, Khan NA, Walochnik J. An update on Acanthamoeba keratitis: diagnosis, pathogenesis and treatment. Parasite. 2015;22:10.

[89] Kumar R, Lloyd D. Recent advances in the treatment of Acanthamoeba keratitis. Clinical Infectious Diseases: An Official Publication of the Infectious Diseases Society of America. 2002;35(4):434-41.

[90] Grayson M. Chagas disease. Nature. 2010;465(7301):S3.

[91] Coura JR, Borges-Pereira J. Chagas disease: 100 years after its discovery. A systemic review. Acta Tropica. 2010;115(1-2):5-13.

[92] Frohlich SJ, Mino de Kaspar H, Peran R, Vera de Bilbao N, Schinini A, Rojas de Arias A, et al. Intraocular involvement of Chagas disease (American trypanosomiasis). Studies in Paraguay/South America. Der Ophthalmologe: Zeitschrift der Deutschen Ophthalmologischen Gesellschaft. 1997;94(3):206-10.

[93] Frohlich SJ, Mino de Kaspar H, Peran R, Rojas de Arias A, Sanchez Insfran N, Moreno Azorero R, et al. Eye involvement in Chagas disease (American trypanosomiasis). 1996/1997 studies in Paraguay. Der Ophthalmologe: Zeitschrift der Deutschen Ophthalmologischen Gesellschaft. 1998;95(3):168-71.

[94] Bern C. Chagas' disease. The New England Journal of Medicine. 2015;373(5):456-66.

[95] Morillo CA, Marin-Neto JA, Avezum A, Sosa-Estani S, Rassi A, Jr., Rosas F, et al. Randomized trial of benznidazole for chronic Chagas' cardiomyopathy. The New England Journal of Medicine. 2015;373(14):1295-306.

[96] Chagas disease. Available at http://www.nytimes.com/health/guides/disease/chagas-disease/overview.html

[97] Leishmaniasis. Available at: http://www.who.int/mediacentre/factsheets/fs375/en/

[98] Badri Prasad B, Shakya A, Poonam L, Smriti K. Caruncular Leishmaniasis – an unusual case. Orbit. 2015;34(4):232-3.

[99] Philips CA, Kalal CR, Kumar KN, Bihari C, Sarin SK. Simultaneous occurrence of ocular, disseminated mucocutaneous, and multivisceral involvement of leishmaniasis. Case Reports in Infectious Diseases. 2014;2014:837625.

[100] Khalil EA, Musa AM, Younis BM, Elfaki ME, Zijlstra EE, Elhassan AM. Blindness following visceral leishmaniasis: a neglected post-kala-azar complication. Tropical Doctor. 2011;41(3):139-40.

[101] Veraldi S, Bottini S, Curro N, Gianotti R. Leishmaniasis of the eyelid mimicking an infundibular cyst and review of the literature on ocular leishmaniasis. International Journal of Infectious Diseases: IJID: Official Publication of the International Society for Infectious Diseases. 2010;14(Suppl 3):e230-2.

[102] Salvanos P, Kabanarou SA, Xirou T, Kourentis C, Feretis E. Proliferative vitreoretinopathy in a child with visceral leishmaniasis. European Journal of Ophthalmology. 2010;20(1):231-3.

[103] Sadeghian G, Nilfroushzadeh MA, Moradi SH, Hanjani SH. Ocular leishmaniasis: a case report. Dermatology Online Journal. 2005;11(2):19.

[104] el-Hassan AM, el-Sheikh EA, Eltoum IA, Ghalib HW, Ali MS, Zijlstra E, et al. Post-kala-azar anterior uveitis: demonstration of Leishmania parasites in the lesion. Transactions of the Royal Society of Tropical Medicine and Hygiene. 1991;85(4):471-3.

[105] Dechant W, Rees PH, Kager PA, Klauss V, Adala H. Post kala-azar uveitis. The British Journal of Ophthalmology. 1980;64(9):680-3.

[106] De Cock KM, Rees PH, Klauss V, Kasili EG, Kager PA, Schattenkerk JK. Retinal hemorrhages in kala-azar. The American Journal of Tropical Medicine and Hygiene. 1982;31(5):927-30.

[107] Montero JA, Ruiz-Moreno JM, Sanchis E. Intraretinal hemorrhage associated with leishmaniasis. Ophthalmic Surgery, Lasers & Imaging: The Official Journal of the International Society for Imaging in the Eye. 2003;34(3):212-4.

[108] Biswas J, Mani B, Bhende M. Spontaneous resolution of bilateral macular haemorrhage in a patient with kala-azar. Eye. 2000;14(Pt 2):244-6.

[109] Mookerjee GC, Sen G, Chaudhuri MD, Chakraborty K. Acute kala-azar with haemorrhagic retinopathy. Journal of the Indian Medical Association. 1975;65(3):86-8.

[110] Maude RJ, Ahmed BU, Rahman AH, Rahman R, Majumder MI, Menezes DB, et al. Retinal changes in visceral leishmaniasis by retinal photography. BMC Infectious Diseases. 2014;14:527.

[111] Oliveira-Neto MP, Martins VJ, Mattos MS, Pirmez C, Brahin LR, Benchimol E. South American cutaneous leishmaniasis of the eyelids: report of five cases in Rio de Janeiro State, Brazil. Ophthalmology. 2000;107(1):169-72.

[112] Chaudhry IA, Hylton C, DesMarchais B. Bilateral ptosis and lower eyelid ectropion secondary to cutaneous leishmaniasis. Archives of Ophthalmology. 1998;116(9):1244-5.

[113] Yaghoobi R, Maraghi S, Bagherani N, Rafiei A. Cutaneous leishmaniasis of the lid: a report of nine cases. Korean Journal of Ophthalmology: KJO. 2010;24(1):40-3.

[114] Baddini-Caramelli C, Matayoshi S, Moura EM, Araf D, Santo R, Voegels R, et al. Chronic dacryocystitis in American mucocutaneous leishmaniasis. Ophthalmic Plastic and Reconstructive Surgery. 2001;17(1):48-52.

[115] Ferrari TC, Guedes AC, Orefice F, Genaro O, Pinheiro SR, Marra MA, et al. Isolation of Leishmania sp. from aqueous humor of a patient with cutaneous disseminated leishmaniasis and bilateral iridocyclitis (preliminary report). Revista do Instituto de Medicina Tropical de Sao Paulo. 1990;32(4):296-8.

[116] Petersen CA, Greenlee MH. Neurologic Manifestations of Leishmania spp. Infection. Journal of Neuroparasitology. 2011;2:N110401.

[117] Ozdemir Y, Kulacoglu S, Cosar CB, Onder F, Kural G. Ocular leishmaniasis. Eye. 1999;13(Pt 5):666-7.

[118] el Hassan AM, Khalil EA, el Sheikh EA, Zijlstra EE, Osman A, Ibrahim ME. Post kala-azar ocular leishmaniasis. Transactions of the Royal Society of Tropical Medicine and Hygiene. 1998;92(2):177-9.

[119] Leite RS, Souza NA, Barbosa AD, Ferreira AL, de Andrade AS. Evaluation of conjunctival swab as a mass-screening tool for molecular diagnosis of canine visceral leishmaniasis. Parasitology Research. 2015;114(6):2255-62.

[120] Shirian S, Oryan A, Hatam GR, Panahi S, Daneshbod Y. Comparison of conventional, molecular, and immunohistochemical methods in diagnosis of typical and atypical cutaneous leishmaniasis. Archives of Pathology & Laboratory Medicine. 2014;138(2): 235-40.

[121] Abrishami M, Soheilian M, Farahi A, Dowlati Y. Successful treatment of ocular leishmaniasis. European Journal of Dermatology: EJD. 2002;12(1):88-9.

[122] Zadeh MM, Manshai K, Shaddel M, Oormazdi H. Ocular leishmaniasis. Iranian Journal of Opthalmology. 2006;19(3):1-5.

[123] World Malaria Report. 2014 (Available at: http://www.who.int/malaria/publications/world_malaria_report_2014/en/).

[124] Sherwood JA. Progess toward understanding the pathogenesis of sequestration in falciparum malaria. Blood Cells. 1990;16(2-3):620-8.

[125] Sherwood JA, Roberts DD, Spitalnik SL, Marsh K, Harvey EB, Miller LH, et al. Parasitized erythrocyte antigens and thrombospondin adhesion in the immunology and pathogenesis of falciparum malaria. Transactions of the Association of American Physicians. 1986;99:206-13.

[126] Lagraulet J, Robet C, Bard J. The ocular complications of malaria. Bulletin de la Société de pathologie exotique. 1967;60(3):217-21.

[127] Bhattacharjya BP, Guha GS. Ocular manifestations in malaria. Indian Medical Gazette. 1946;81:79.

[128] Ross JV. Ocular complications associated with malaria. Eye Ear Nose Throat Monthly. 1953;32(12):707-11.

[129] Schemann JF, Doumbo O, Malvy D, Traore L, Kone A, Sidibe T, et al. Ocular lesions associated with malaria in children in Mali. The American Journal of Tropical Medicine and Hygiene. 2002;67(1):61-3.

[130] Maude RJ, Hassan MU, Beare NA. Severe retinal whitening in an adult with cerebral malaria. The American Journal of Tropical Medicine and Hygiene. 2009;80(6):881.

[131] Looareesuwan S, Warrell DA, White NJ, Chanthavanich P, Warrell MJ, Chantaratherakitti S, et al. Retinal hemorrhage, a common sign of prognostic significance in cere-

bral malaria. The American Journal of Tropical Medicine and Hygiene. 1983;32(5): 911-5.

[132] Beare NA, Taylor TE, Harding SP, Lewallen S, Molyneux ME. Malarial retinopathy: a newly established diagnostic sign in severe malaria. The American Journal of Tropical Medicine and Hygiene. 2006;75(5):790-7.

[133] Wongsrichanalai C, Barcus MJ, Muth S, Sutamihardja A, Wernsdorfer WH. A review of malaria diagnostic tools: microscopy and rapid diagnostic test (RDT). The American Journal of Tropical Medicine and Hygiene. 2007;77(6 Suppl):119-27.

[134] Hidayat AA, Nalbandian RM, Sammons DW, Fleischman JA, Johnson TE. The diagnostic histopathologic features of ocular malaria. Ophthalmology. 1993;100(8):1183-6.

[135] Lewallen S, Taylor TE, Molyneux ME, Wills BA, Courtright P. Ocular fundus findings in Malawian children with cerebral malaria. Ophthalmology. 1993;100(6):857-61.

[136] Nwosu S. Ocular complications of malaria treatment. Nigerian Journal of Clinical Practice. 2012;15(1):95-7.

[137] Beare NA, Southern C, Chalira C, Taylor TE, Molyneux ME, Harding SP. Prognostic significance and course of retinopathy in children with severe malaria. Archives of Ophthalmology. 2004;122(8):1141-7.

[138] Keeling P. Five questions about microsporidia. PLoS Pathogens. 2009;5(9):e1000489.

[139] Lowder CY, McMahon JT, Meisler DM, Dodds EM, Calabrese LH, Didier ES, et al. Microsporidial keratoconjunctivitis caused by Septata intestinalis in a patient with acquired immunodeficiency syndrome. American Journal of Ophthalmology. 1996;121(6):715-7.

[140] Shadduck JA, Meccoli RA, Davis R, Font RL. Isolation of a microsporidian from a human patient. The Journal of Infectious Diseases. 1990;162(3):773-6.

[141] Diesenhouse MC, Wilson LA, Corrent GF, Visvesvara GS, Grossniklaus HE, Bryan RT. Treatment of microsporidial keratoconjunctivitis with topical fumagillin. American Journal of Ophthalmology. 1993;115(3):293-8.

[142] Das S, Wallang BS, Sharma S, Bhadange YV, Balne PK, Sahu SK. The efficacy of corneal debridement in the treatment of microsporidial keratoconjunctivitis: a prospective randomized clinical trial. American Journal of Ophthalmology. 2014;157(6): 1151-5.

[143] Sanjay S. Clinical trial of 0.02% polyhexamethylene biguanide versus placebo in the treatment of microsporidial keratoconjunctivitis. American Journal of Ophthalmology. 2011;151(1):183.

[144] Savioli L, Smith H, Thompson A. Giardia and Cryptosporidium join the "Neglected Diseases Initiative'. Trends in Parasitology. 2006;22(5):203-8.

[145] Halliez MC, Buret AG. Extra-intestinal and long term consequences of Giardia duodenalis infections. World Journal of Gastroenterology. 2013;19(47):8974-85.

[146] Corsi A, Nucci C, Knafelz D, Bulgarini D, Di Iorio L, Polito A, et al. Ocular changes associated with Giardia lamblia infection in children. The British Journal of Ophthalmology. 1998;82(1):59-62.

[147] Gardner TB, Hill DR. Treatment of giardiasis. Clinical Microbiology Reviews. 2001;14(1):114-28.

[148] Onchocerciasis. (Available: http://www.who.int/mediacentre/factsheets/fs374/en/).

[149] Udall DN. Recent updates on onchocerciasis: diagnosis and treatment. Clinical Infectious Diseases: An Official Publication of the Infectious Diseases Society of America. 2007;44(1):53-60.

[150] Parasites – Onchocerciasis. (Available at: http://www.cdc.gov/parasites/onchocerciasis/epi.html).

[151] Hall LR, Pearlman E. Pathogenesis of onchocercal keratitis (River blindness). Clinical Microbiology Reviews. 1999;12(3):445-53.

[152] Higazi TB, Filiano A, Katholi CR, Dadzie Y, Remme JH, Unnasch TR. Wolbachia endosymbiont levels in severe and mild strains of Onchocerca volvulus. Molecular and Biochemical Parasitology. 2005;141(1):109-12.

[153] Brattig NW. Pathogenesis and host responses in human onchocerciasis: impact of Onchocerca filariae and Wolbachia endobacteria. Microbes and Infection. 2004;6(1):113-28.

[154] Tamarozzi F, Halliday A, Gentil K, Hoerauf A, Pearlman E, Taylor MJ. Onchocerciasis: the role of Wolbachia bacterial endosymbionts in parasite biology, disease pathogenesis, and treatment. Clinical Microbiology Reviews. 2011;24(3):459-68.

[155] Harnett W. DNA-based detection of onchocerca volvulus. Transactions of the Royal Society of Tropical Medicine and Hygiene. 2002;96(Suppl 1):S231-4.

[156] Boatin BA, Toe L, Alley ES, Nagelkerke NJ, Borsboom G, Habbema JD. Detection of Onchocerca volvulus infection in low prevalence areas: a comparison of three diagnostic methods. Parasitology. 2002;125(Pt 6):545-52.

[157] Pischke S, Buttner DW, Liebau E, Fischer P. An internal control for the detection of Onchocerca volvulus DNA by PCR-ELISA and rapid detection of specific PCR products by DNA Detection Test Strips. Tropical Medicine & International Health. 2002;7(6):526-31.

[158] Ayong LS, Tume CB, Wembe FE, Simo G, Asonganyi T, Lando G, et al. Development and evaluation of an antigen detection dipstick assay for the diagnosis of human onchocerciasis. Tropical Medicine & International Health. 2005;10(3):228-33.

[159] Nde PN, Pogonka T, Bradley JE, Titanji VP, Lucius R. Sensitive and specific serodiagnosis of onchocerciasis with recombinant hybrid proteins. The American Journal of Tropical Medicine and Hygiene. 2002;66(5):566-71.

[160] Onchocerciasis. Available at http://www.cdc.gov/parasites/onchocerciasis/

[161] Onchocerciasis. (Available at: http://www.cdc.gov/parasites/onchocerciasis/health_professionals/).

[162] Parasites – Loiasis. (Available at: http://www.cdc.gov/parasites/loiasis/epi.html).

[163] Kelly-Hope LA, Bockarie MJ, Molyneux DH. Loa loa ecology in central Africa: role of the Congo River system. PLoS Neglected Tropical Diseases. 2012;6(6):e1605.

[164] Bhedasgaonkar S, Baile RB, Nadkarni S, Jakkula G, Gogri P. Loa loa macrofilariasis in the eyelid: case report of the first periocular subcutaneous manifestation in India. Journal of Parasitic Diseases. 2011;35(2):230-1.

[165] Cho HY, Lee YJ, Shin SY, Song HO, Ahn MH, Ryu JS. Subconjuctival Loa loa with Calabar swelling. Journal of Korean Medical Science. 2008;23(4):731-3.

[166] Dupont A, Zue-N'dong J, Pinder M. Common occurrence of amicrofilaraemic Loa loa filariasis within the endemic region. Transactions of the Royal Society of Tropical Medicine and Hygiene. 1988;82(5):730.

[167] Geldelman D, Blumberg R, Sadun A. Ocular Loa loa with cryoprobe extraction of subconjunctival worm. Ophthalmology. 1984;91(3):300-3.

[168] Klion AD, Vijaykumar A, Oei T, Martin B, Nutman TB. Serum immunoglobulin G4 antibodies to the recombinant antigen, Ll-SXP-1, are highly specific for Loa loa infection. The Journal of Infectious Diseases. 2003;187(1):128-33.

[169] Boussinesq M. Loiasis. Annals of Tropical Medicine and Parasitology. 2006;100(8):715-31.

[170] Loiasis. Available at: http://www.cdc.gov/parasites/loiasis/treatment.html (Accessed on 30 March 2016).

[171] Kalogeropoulos CD, Stefaniotou MI, Gorgoli KE, Papadopoulou CV, Pappa CN, Paschidis CA. Ocular dirofilariasis: a case series of 8 patients. Middle East African Journal of Ophthalmology. 2014;21(4):312-6.

[172] Sahdev SI, Sureka SP, Sathe PA, Agashe R. Ocular dirofilariasis: still in the dark in western India? Journal of Postgraduate Medicine. 2012;58(3):227-8.

[173] Sekhar HS, Srinivasa H, Batru RR, Mathai E, Shariff S, Macaden RS. Human ocular dirofilariasis in Kerala Southern India. Indian Journal of Pathology & Microbiology. 2000;43(1):77-9.

[174] Font RL, Neafie RC, Perry HD. Subcutaneous dirofilariasis of the eyelid and ocular adnexa. Report of six cases. Archives of Ophthalmology. 1980;98(6):1079-82.

[175] Gorezis S, Psilla M, Asproudis I, Peschos D, Papadopoulou C, Stefaniotou M. Intravitreal dirofilariasis: a rare ocular infection. Orbit. 2006;25(1):57-9.

[176] Perera L, Perez-Arellano JL, Cordero M, Simon F, Muro A. Utility of antibodies against a 22 kD molecule of Dirofilaria immitis in the diagnosis of human pulmonary dirofilariasis. Tropical Medicine & International Health. 1998;3(2):151-5.

[177] Dirofilariasis. Available at: http://www.cdc.gov/parasites/dirofilariasis/faqs.html (Accessed 0n 30 March 2016).

[178] Mittal M, Sathish KR, Bhatia PG, Chidamber BS. Ocular dirofilariasis in Dubai, UAE. Indian Journal of Ophthalmology. 2008;56(4):325-6.

[179] Diaz JH. Gnathostomiasis: an emerging infection of raw fish consumers in Gnathostoma nematode-endemic and nonendemic countries. Journal of Travel Medicine. 2015;22(5):318-24.

[180] Wiwanitkit V. Gnathostomiasis and sushi ingestion. American Journal of Dermatopathology. 2012;34(6):675.

[181] Sujata DN, Renu BS. Intraocular gnathostomiasis from coastal part of Maharashtra. Tropical Parasitology. 2013;3(1):82-4.

[182] Pillai GS, Kumar A, Radhakrishnan N, Maniyelil J, Shafi T, Dinesh KR, et al. Intraocular gnathostomiasis: report of a case and review of literature. The American Journal of Tropical Medicine and Hygiene. 2012;86(4):620-3.

[183] Bhattacharjee H, Das D, Medhi J. Intravitreal gnathostomiasis and review of literature. Retina. 2007;27(1):67-73.

[184] Buppajarntham A, Apisarnthanarak A, Khawcharoenporn T, Rutjanawech S, Mundy LM. Asymptomatic eosinophilia due to gnathostomiasis. International Journal of Infectious Diseases: IJID: Official Publication of the International Society for Infectious Diseases. 2014;23:14-5.

[185] Saksirisampant W, Chawengkiattikul R, Kraivichain K, Nuchprayoon S. Specific IgE antibody responses to somatic and excretory-secretory antigens of third stage G. spinigerum larvae in human gnathostomiasis. Journal of the Medical Association of Thailand. 2001;84(Suppl 1):S173-81.

[186] Saenseeha S, Penchom J, Yamasaki H, Laummaunwai P, Tayapiwatana C, Kitkhuandee A, et al. A dot-ELISA test using a Gnathostoma spinigerum recombinant matrix metalloproteinase protein for the serodiagnosis of human gnathostomiasis. The Southeast Asian Journal of Tropical Medicine and Public health. 2014;45(5):990-6.

[187] Laummaunwai P, Sawanyawisuth K, Intapan PM, Chotmongkol V, Wongkham C, Maleewong W. Evaluation of human IgG class and subclass antibodies to a 24 kDa antigenic component of Gnathostoma spinigerum for the serodiagnosis of gnathostomiasis. Parasitology Research. 2007;101(3):703-8.

[188] Herman JS, Chiodini PL. Gnathostomiasis, another emerging imported disease. Clinical Microbiology Reviews. 2009;22(3):484-92.

[189] Anantaphruti MT. ELISA for diagnosis of gnathostomiasis using antigens from Gnathostoma doloresi and G. spinigerum. The Southeast Asian Journal of Tropical Medicine and Public Health. 1989;20(2):297-304.

[190] Maleewong W, Morakote N, Thamasonthi W, Charuchinda K, Tesana S, Khamboonruang C. Serodiagnosis of human gnathostomiasis. The Southeast Asian Journal of Tropical Medicine and Public Health. 1988;19(2):201-5.

[191] Nawa Y, Katchanov J, Yoshikawa M, Rojekittikhun W, Dekumyoy P, Kusolusuk T, et al. Ocular Gnathostomiasis: a comprehensive review. J Trop Med Parasitol. 2010;33:77-86.

[192] Joseph A, Joseph A. Ocular thelaziasis (a case report). Indian Journal of Ophthalmology. 1985;33(2):113-4.

[193] Yospaiboon Y, Sithithavorn P, Maleewong V, Ukosanakarn U, Bhaibulaya M. Ocular thelaziasis in Thailand: a case report. Journal of the Medical Association of Thailand. 1989;72(8):469-73.

[194] Thelaziasis. Available at: http://www.cdc.gov/dpdx/thelaziasis/tx.html

[195] Jee D, Kim KS, Lee WK, Kim W, Jeon S. Clinical features of ocular toxocariasis in adult Korean patients. Ocular Immunology and Inflammation. 2016;24(2):207-16.

[196] Yokoi K, Goto H, Sakai J, Usui M. Clinical features of ocular toxocariasis in Japan. Ocular Immunology and Inflammation. 2003;11(4):269-75.

[197] Zhou M, Chang Q, Gonzales JA, Chen Q, Zhang Y, Huang X, et al. Clinical characteristics of ocular toxocariasis in Eastern China. Graefe's archive for clinical and experimental ophthalmology = Albrecht von Graefes Archiv fur klinische und experimentelle Ophthalmologie. 2012;250(9):1373-8.

[198] Woodhall D, Starr MC, Montgomery SP, Jones JL, Lum F, Read RW, et al. Ocular toxocariasis: epidemiologic, anatomic, and therapeutic variations based on a survey of ophthalmic subspecialists. Ophthalmology. 2012;119(6):1211-7.

[199] Centers for Disease C, Prevention. Ocular toxocariasis – United States, 2009-2010. MMWR Morbidity and Mortality Weekly Report. 2011;60(22):734-6.

[200] Ahn SJ, Ryoo NK, Woo SJ. Ocular toxocariasis: clinical features, diagnosis, treatment, and prevention. Asia Pacific Allergy. 2014;4(3):134-41.

[201] Arevalo JF, Espinoza JV, Arevalo FA. Ocular toxocariasis. Journal of Pediatric Ophthalmology and Strabismus. 2013;50(2):76-86.

[202] Ament CS, Young LH. Ocular manifestations of helminthic infections: onchocersiasis, cysticercosis, toxocariasis, and diffuse unilateral subacute neuroretinitis. International Ophthalmology Clinics. 2006;46(2):1-10.

[203] Teyssot N, Cassoux N, Lehoang P, Bodaghi B. Fuchs heterochromic cyclitis and ocular toxocariasis. American Journal of Ophthalmology. 2005;139(5):915-6.

[204] Stewart JM, Cubillan LD, Cunningham ET, Jr. Prevalence, clinical features, and causes of vision loss among patients with ocular toxocariasis. Retina. 2005;25(8):1005-13.

[205] Martinez-Pulgarin DF, Munoz-Urbano M, Gomez-Suta LD, Delgado OM, Rodriguez-Morales AJ. Ocular toxocariasis: new diagnostic and therapeutic perspectives. Recent Patents on Anti-Infective Drug Discovery. 2015;10(1):35-41.

[206] Lee TH, Ji YS, Lee SH. ELISA-confirmed bilateral ocular toxocariasis with different features. Optometry and Vision Science: Official Publication of the American Academy of Optometry. 2015;92(8):e176-9.

[207] Schneier AJ, Durand ML. Ocular toxocariasis: advances in diagnosis and treatment. International Ophthalmology Clinics. 2011;51(4):135-44.

[208] de Visser L, Rothova A, de Boer JH, van Loon AM, Kerkhoff FT, Canninga-van Dijk MR, et al. Diagnosis of ocular toxocariasis by establishing intraocular antibody production. American Journal of Ophthalmology. 2008;145(2):369-74.

[209] Jacquier P, Gottstein B, Stingelin Y, Eckert J. Immunodiagnosis of toxocarosis in humans: evaluation of a new enzyme-linked immunosorbent assay kit. Journal of Clinical Microbiology. 1991;29(9):1831-5.

[210] Jin Y, Shen C, Huh S, Sohn WM, Choi MH, Hong ST. Serodiagnosis of toxocariasis by ELISA using crude antigen of Toxocara canis larvae. The Korean Journal of Parasitology. 2013;51(4):433-9.

[211] Tian JX, O'Hagan S. Toxocara polymerase chain reaction on ocular fluids in bilateral granulomatous chorioretinitis. International Medical Case Reports Journal. 2015;8:107-10.

[212] Van De N, Trung NV, Duyet le V, Chai JY. Molecular diagnosis of an ocular toxocariasis patient in Vietnam. The Korean Journal of Parasitology. 2013;51(5):563-7.

[213] Zibaei M, Sadjjadi SM, Karamian M, Uga S, Oryan A, Jahadi-Hosseini SH. A comparative histopathology, serology and molecular study, on experimental ocular toxocariasis by Toxocara cati in Mongolian gerbils and Wistar rats. BioMed Research International. 2013;2013:109580.

[214] Seong S, Moon D, Lee DK, Kim HE, Oh HS, Kim SH, et al. A case of ocular toxocariasis successfully treated with albendazole and triamcinolon. The Korean Journal of Parasitology. 2014;52(5):537-40.

[215] Frazier M, Anderson ML, Sophocleous S. Treatment of ocular toxocariasis with albendezole: a case report. Optometry. 2009;80(4):175-80.

[216] Prasad KN, Prasad A, Verma A, Singh AK. Human cysticercosis and Indian scenario: a review. Journal of Biosciences. 2008;33(4):571-82.

[217] Coral-Almeida M, Gabriel S, Abatih EN, Praet N, Benitez W, Dorny P. Taenia solium Human Cysticercosis: a systematic review of sero-epidemiological data from endemic zones around the world. PLoS Neglected Tropical Diseases. 2015;9(7):e0003919.

[218] Yera H, Dupont D, Houze S, Ben M'rad M, Pilleux F, Sulahian A, et al. Confirmation and follow-up of neurocysticercosis by real-time PCR in cerebrospinal fluid samples of patients living in France. Journal of Clinical Microbiology. 2011;49(12):4338-40.

[219] Jain RS, Kumar S, Bhana I, Agarwal R. Ocular cysticercosis with vitreous hemorrhage: a rare complication of a common disease. Springerplus. 2015;4:217.

[220] Goyal S, Sandhu PS, Sharma A, Malik MA, Bansal P, Kaur J. Inferior rectus muscle ocular cysticercosis: a case report. Saudi Journal of Ophthalmology. 2015;29(2):175-7.

[221] Mohan N, Panda KG, Padhi TR. Bug inside the eye: ocular cysticercosis. JAMA Ophthalmology. 2014;132(12):1468.

[222] Sohoni CA. Neuro-ocular cysticercosis causing total retinal detachment and cataract. Journal of Family Medicine and Primary Care. 2013;2(3):300-1.

[223] Labh RK, Sharma AK. Ptosis: a rare presentation of ocular cysticercosis. Nepalese Journal of Ophthalmology. 2013;5(1):133-5.

[224] Sharma AK. Ocular cysticercosis: diagnosis and treatment. Nepalese Journal of Ophthalmology. 2014;6(2):240-1.

[225] Nkouawa A, Sako Y, Nakao M, Nakaya K, Ito A. Loop-mediated isothermal amplification method for differentiation and rapid detection of Taenia species. Journal of Clinical Microbiology. 2009;47(1):168-74.

[226] Swastika K, Dewiyani CI, Yanagida T, Sako Y, Sudarmaja M, Sutisna P, et al. An ocular cysticercosis in Bali, Indonesia caused by Taenia solium Asian genotype. Parasitology International. 2012;61(2):378-80.

[227] Ocular cysticercosis treatment and management. Available at: http://emedcine.medscape.com/article/1204683-treatment

[228] Stojkovic M, Junghanss T. Cystic and alveolar echinococcosis. Handbook of Clininical Neurology. 2013;114:327-34.

[229] Karakas HM, Tokoglu F, Kacar M, Boyacigil S. Retrobulbar hydatid cyst: assessment of two cases. Australasian Radiology. 1997;41(2):179-80.

[230] Budke CM, Carabin H, Ndimubanzi PC, Nguyen H, Rainwater E, Dickey M, et al. A systematic review of the literature on cystic echinococcosis frequency worldwide and

its associated clinical manifestations. The American Journal of Tropical Medicine and Hygiene. 2013;88(6):1011-27.

[231] Arora MM, Dhanda RP, Bhagwat AG, Kalevar VK. Intra-ocular hydatid cyst. The British Journal of Ophthalmology. 1964;48:507-9.

[232] Betharia SM, Sharma V, Pushker N. Ultrasound findings in orbital hydatid cysts. American Journal of Ophthalmology. 2003;135(4):568-70.

[233] Aksoy FG, Tanrikulu S, Kosar U. Inferiorly located retrobulbar hydatid cyst: CT and MRI features. Computerized Medical Imaging and Graphics. 2001;25(6):535-40.

[234] Manzano-Roman R, Sanchez-Ovejero C, Hernandez-Gonzalez A, Casulli A, Siles-Lucas M. Serological diagnosis and follow-up of human cystic echinococcosis: a new hope for the future? BioMed Research international. 2015;2015:428205.

[235] Mirfazaelian H, Bagheri B, Daneshbod Y. Fine needle aspiration cytology diagnosis of an ocular hydatid cyst. Cytopathology. 2014;25(6):416-7.

[236] Echinococcosis. Available at: http://www.cfsph.iastate.edu/Factsheets/pdfs/echinococcosis.pdf

[237] Al-Muala HD, Sami SM, Shukri MA, Hasson HK, Alaboudy AT. Orbital hydatid cyst. Annals of Maxillofacial Surgery. 2012;2(2):197-9.

[238] Selcuklu A, Ozturk M, Kulahli I, Dogan H. Successful surgical management of an intraorbital hydatid cyst through a transmaxillary approach: case report. Skull Base: Official Journal of North American Skull Base Society. 2003;13(2):101-5.

[239] Mas-Coma S, Agramunt VH, Valero MA. Neurological and ocular fascioliasis in humans. Advances in Parasitology. 2014;84:27-149.

[240] Dickinson AJ, Rosenthal AR, Nicholson KG. Inflammation of the retinal pigment epithelium: a unique presentation of ocular schistosomiasis. The British Journal of Ophthalmology. 1990;74(7):440-2.

[241] Mimori T, Hirai H, Kifune T, Inada K. Philophthalmus sp. (Trematoda) in a human eye. The American Journal of Tropical Medicine and Hygiene. 1982;31(4):859-61.

[242] Tiewchaloern S, Udomkijdecha S, Suvouttho S, Chunchamsri K, Waikagul J. Clinostomum trematode from human eye. The Southeast Asian Journal of Tropical Medicine and Public health. 1999;30(2):382-4.

[243] McDonald HR, Kazacos KR, Schatz H, Johnson RN. Two cases of intraocular infection with Alaria mesocercaria (Trematoda). American Journal of Ophthalmology. 1994;117(4):447-55.

[244] Dono M, Bertonati MR, Poggi R, Teneggi E, Maddalo F, Via F, et al. Three cases of ophthalmomyiasis externa by sheep botfly Oestrus ovis in Italy. New Microbiologica. 2005;28(4):365-8.

[245] Grammer J, Erb C, Kamin G, Wild M, Riedinger C, Kosmidis P, et al. Ophthalmomyiasis externa due to the sheep botfly Oestrus ovis (Diptera: Oestridae) in southwest Germany. German Journal of Ophthalmology. 1995;4(3):188-95.

[246] Gupta VP, Baveja UK. Ophthalmomyiasis externa caused by the sheep nasal botfly Oestrus ovis. Indian Journal of Ophthalmology. 1988;36(1):41-2.

[247] Harvey JT. Sheep botfly: ophthalmomyiasis externa. Canadian Journal of Ophthalmology (Journal canadien d'ophtalmologie). 1986;21(3):92-5.

[248] Mason GI. Bilateral ophthalmomyiasis interna. American Journal of Ophthalmology. 1981;91(1):65-70.

[249] Ho-Yen DO, Chapman DJ, Ashburn D. Immunoblotting can help the diagnosis of ocular toxoplasmosis. Molecular Pathology. 2000;53(3):155-8.

[250] Fekkar A, Bodaghi B, Touafek F, Le Hoang P, Mazier D, Paris L. Comparison of immunoblotting, calculation of the Goldmann-Witmer coefficient, and real-time PCR using aqueous humor samples for diagnosis of ocular toxoplasmosis. Journal of Clinical Microbiology. 2008;46(6):1965-7.

Chapter 4

Acanthamoeba Keratitis: The Emerging Vision-Threatening Corneal Disease

Lidia Chomicz, Jacek P. Szaflik, Marcin Padzik and Justyna Izdebska

Additional information is available at the end of the chapter

http://dx.doi.org/10.5772/64848

Abstract

Some *Acanthamoeba* species are distributed in natural and man-made environments, in a wide range of soil and aquatic habitats, also in clinical settings. The amphizoic organisms can exist as facultative parasites - causative agents of serious human disease, *Acanthamoeba* keratitis. The vision-threatening eye disease occurring particularly in contact lens wearers is reported with increasing prevalence in different regions of the world. The amoebic keratitis is difficult to diagnose as clinical symptoms are similar to those observed in other eye diseases. Moreover, bacterial, viral, fungal, and amoebic co-infections frequently occur; also amoebae act as carriers for ~ 20 species pathogenic for humans, e.g. from *Pseudomonas, Legionella, Mycobacterium* and *Escherichia* genera; thus the corneal disease is frequently misdiagnosed. Complex etiology, late proper recognition of amoebic infections, and the exceptional resistance of *Acanthamoeba* cysts to chemicals are important factors influencing diagnostic and therapeutic difficulties. Surgical interventions are needed as an alternative treatment in refractory *Acanthamoeba* keratitis. It should be taken into consideration that the knowledge and awareness of increasing threat generated by the amphizoic amoebae are still insufficient. This compilation presents selected aspects of eye disease that is becoming the increasingly significant for human health worldwide.

Keywords: *Acanthamoeba* keratitis, risk factors, symptoms, pathogenesis, diagnostics, therapy

1. Introduction

Acanthamoeba keratitis (AK), the vision-threatening corneal disease that was first time recognized in 1973 in the United States in a Texas rancher [1], is reported with increasing prevalence in different regions and countries year after year [1- 7]. This corneal, usually acute and progressive infection is becoming increasingly significant for human health worldwide.

Eye diseases affecting the cornea are a major cause of blindness worldwide. Among different infectious agents, bacteria, fungi, viruses and protozoans may be causes of keratitis in contact lens users. At present, the epidemiology of microbial keratitis is complicated, diverse, and even controversial; the use of contact lenses is considered as the most important risk factor of corneal infections in humans [4,8]. It was emphasized in several reviews [8- 10] that the incidence rates of particular organisms causing keratitis associated with contact lens wear differ between parts of the world, from country to country and even from one population to another. Economic factors, various frequencies of contact lens wear in particular geographical locations, different availabilities and standards of eye care, and different methods of etiological agent isolation and culture in particular surveys were mentioned as factors influencing the differences and criteria taken into consideration in the studies.

The frequency of microbial keratitis cases caused by Gram-negative bacteria from genus *Pseudomonas* (as percent of total isolates from given location) varied in Europe: from 6.6% in Turkey to 72.2% in Italy and from 12% to 28.5% in various surveys from the United Kingdom [8]. Climate also influenced the incidence of bacterial keratitis: e.g.in Australia, the frequency of *P. aeruginosa* contact lens keratitis was increased in tropical zones than temperate zones.

The highest proportion of fungal corneal infections (*Aspergillus* sp., *Candida* sp.), 67% was found in India [9]; in Europe, the highest frequency of 22.2% was found in Turkey.

Correlations between the contact lens wear and percentages of bacterial and fungal keratitis were statistically significant.

The viruses from *Herpes* spp. are other agents of keratitis. There are relatively few studies on the epidemiology of *Herpes* keratitis in humans. According to review by Farooq and Shukla [11], in developed countries, *Herpes* keratitis is believed to be an important cause of infectious blindness mainly resulting from stromal opacification, e.g. it was reported from France that the incidence was 25.8 (21.2–30.4) per 100,000 person-years; 95% of the cases occurred in contact lens users. These authors found that the incidence of this keratitis is about 1.5 million, including 40,000 new cases of severe visual impairment each year, however, it is difficult to ascertain the frequency of the viral keratitis because of a lack of surveillance-based epidemiologic studies [11].

Protozoan eye disease, *Acanthamoeba* keratitis (AK), is rare in the general population (estimated incidence: 1.4 per million person- year) but much frequent in contact lens wearers. [4,12,13]. In the United States, an estimated 85% of cases occur in contact lens users. The incidence of the disease in developed countries is approximately 1-33 cases per million contact lens wearers, e.g. in England 17-21 cases per million. Currently, it is emphasized that an awareness and knowledge about AK -the serious, vision-threatening eye disease are still insufficient [12,18].

Previous and recent studies continued in many centers with a participation of practicing researchers and other scientists are crucial for a better understanding of *Acanthamoeba* keratitis [4,14-18]. Advances in the field are expected by both laboratory and clinical practitioners; particularly, an improvement in duration from first symptoms until suitable diagnosis as well as in efficacy of the therapeutic management and prophylaxis is the urgent need. Here, we present selected aspects of this multi-factorial human disease, including the results of our studies and own experiences in the topic.

1.1. Possible environmental sources of *Acanthamoeba* spp.

Free-living amoebae belonging to *Acanthamoeba* genus are ubiquitous and widely distributed in natural and man-made environments of many parts of the world [4,19-25]. The amoebae have been isolated from a wide range of soil and aquatic habitats; they occur in sea, fresh-chlorinated- and tap- water, drinking water systems, bottled mineral water, thermal recreational waters, swimming pools, air, air-conditioning systems including humidifiers, soil and dust, and sewage. The amoeboid protists have been found in fruits, vegetables, and also healthy, diseased or dead animals [12,18]. The amoebae have been isolated also from clinical settings and the hospital environment: on surfaces of different equipment and accessories, in water and air-conditioning systems, on surgical instruments, in dental irrigation units, in contact lenses and their cases, and in dialyzers [7,26,27].

1.2. The developmental forms and classification of *Acanthamoeba* spp.

The amoeboid, mitochondria-bearing protist is known as free-living organism that exists in two morphologic forms: trophozoite and cyst [4,12,18]. The life cycle of *Acanthamoeba* is asexual; the reproduction of trophozoite is by binary fission. This active vegetative stage contains one nucleus with large, central nucleolus (endosome), ectoplasm and granular endoplasm, with a large contractile vacuole as well as numerous mitochondria and digestive vacuoles. The trophozoite is changing in shape, 15–45μm in size and moving by cytoplasmic-transparent pseudopodia that create characteristic protrusions: spine-like acanthopodia. The dormant stage, cyst is smaller, 8-24μm in size, rounded or polygonal in shape, and double - walled, with wrinkled or rippled outer layer; the form indicates minimal metabolic activity. The outer wall of the cyst, the so-called ectocyst, contains lipids and proteins; the inner cyst wall, endocyst contains cellulose that is not present in trophozoite stage. The two cyst walls are separated by a space, except of points in that both walls meet; in these points - pores, i.e. ostioles occur that are covered by plugs, so-called opercula. The plugs are removed when trophozoites emerge from cysts during excystation [4,12]. Trophozoites transform into cyst stages after the growth developmental phase of amoeba population, in which high cell density occurs as well as under harmful environmental conditions (e.g. extremes in temperature and pH, increased or decreased osmolarity, lack of nutrients). The therapeutic experience and many *in vitro* studies showed that the cysts are highly resistant to antimicrobial drugs and a variety of chemical and physical agents [reviewed in 4,12]; they can remain viable under prolonged desiccation, starvation, heat and cold. Also, they can survive *in vitro* in distilled water as long as 25 years [28] and maintain their viability and virulence.

Following the recognition of the amoebae and increasing number of isolates belonging to the genus *Acanthamoeba*, for years they were classified using morphological criteria. In this classification, a size of cysts and the number of characteristic arm -like structures visible within a single cyst in light microscope were mainly taken into consideration [4,12,18,29,30]. At the time, 18 species have been determined and placed in three morphological groups I, II and III.

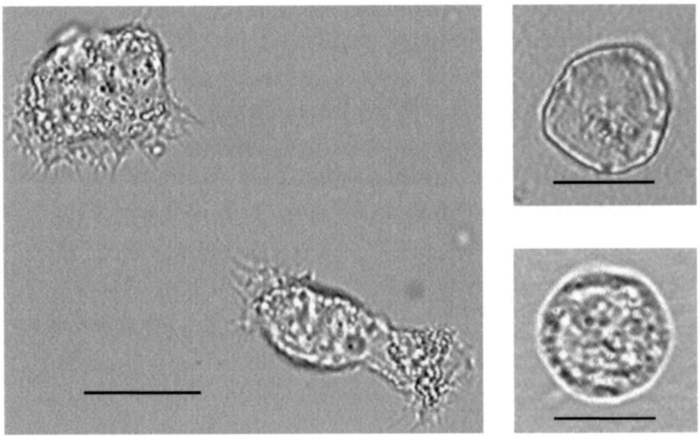

Figure 1. *Acanthamoeba* sp. - wet-mount slides from corneal scrapings; note characteristic spine-like acanthopodia in trophozoites and the double-walled cysts; light micrographs; scale bar = 10μm

The classification of *Acanthamoeba* species /isolates changed with the advances in molecular methods. Recently, it is based on genotype associations - the 18S rRNA gene sequence [5,20,31-33]. The modern approach differs from morphology solely: the species identification is based on combination of the morphological and molecular characterization [3,5,15,20]. At present, 18 or19 genotypes are distinguished for diagnostics and for the characterization of clinical and environmental *Acanthamoeba* isolates [12,15,18,31-33].

2. *Acanthamoeba* spp. as potential agents of human diseases

The protozoans belonging to *Acanthamoeba* spp. complete their life cycles in different outer environments as free-living organisms. Trophozoite forms are able to feed on various micro-organisms dwelling in soil and water (on bacteria, algae, and yeasts as well as on other protozoans) and on small organic particles. In natural, and even in man-made environments, the amoebae develop without entering human or animal organisms. However, in predisposing circumstances, the amoebae may enter the human body. According to literature [34,35], there are evidences from various regions that humans are exposed frequently to the amoebae: it has been confirmed by 50–100% of the healthy populations having specific anti- *Acanthamoeba* antibodies. The protists may permeate into the human body without pathogenic consequences. Investigations in which serological, biochemical and molecular methods were applied showed that people may be exposed both, to pathogenic as well as non-pathogenic *Acanthamoeba* strains [reviewed in 12,13,18]. In immunocompetent individuals, infections with these amoebae may be asymptomatic and/or self-limited.

Nevertheless, several amoebic strains belonging to this genus are able to enter, and colonize human organs and multiply within them, indicating pathogenic effects [4,12,26,27,36].

http://dx.doi.org/10.5772/64848

For this reason, these amoebae are called amphizoic amoebae, because they are able to exist in two different modes: as free-living-exozoic organisms and as endozoic parasitic organisms, within host tissues; thus, the free-living protozoans are also believed as facultative parasites.

Trophozoites and cysts of *Acanthamoeba* were detected during infections of various human cavities and tissues: in paranasal sinuses in rhino-sinusitis, in skin inflammation and skin ulceration, and in pneumonia [7,37,38]. We also found trophozoites and numerous cysts of *Acanthamoeba* among the oral cavity microbiota in 4% somatically and mentally disordered patients. The amoebae accompanied infections with other amoebae, *Entamoeba gingivalis*, the oral amoebae associated with a prolonged deterioration of the periodontium and gingiva [39].

Developmental stages of the amphizoic species may be causative agents of an systemic opportunistic disease developing in immunocompromised individuals. This is rare but almost always fatal granulomatous *Acanthamoeba* encephalitis (GAE) [6,12,18,40]. Other infection caused by the amphizoic amoebae may result in a sight-threatening *Acanthamoeba* keratitis (AK), a non-opportunistic disease occurring mainly in immunocompetent persons, mostly in contact lens wearers [1-3,7,14].

3. Pathogenesis in AK

In the early phase of AK, there are nonspecific symptoms variable in their intensity starting with redness, photophobia, and excessive tearing. Most commonly, only one eye is involved. Active epithelial inflammations usually progress from the outermost layer of the cornea deeper, to the stroma. Symptoms of the devastating eye disease include loss of the visual acuity. In many cases of AK, excruciating eye pain occurs, in which the intensity is often incommensurate with relatively small degree of corneal deterioration. There are clinical and histopathological evidences that the severe pain is associated with *Acanthamoeba* trophozoite activeness that result in the inflammation of the corneal nerves -radial keratoneuritis [4,27]. It is also emphasized that a characteristic ring-like corneal infiltration may occur in some patients. This amoebic eye infection may develop from a few days to several months, as a severe, prolonged disease, which, without suitable treatment may lead to blindness.

A pathogenesis of *Acanthamoeba* keratitis is a multi-factorial process connected with some factors contributing directly and indirectly in production of diseases in humans [12].

Among the direct contributing factors, the following are listed: adhesion of *Acanthamoeba* trophozoites to host cells, phagocytosis to take up food particles, neuraminidase activity, and secretion of toxins. The neuraminidase enzyme, which is active at 25-30 ºC, is believed to be important in a damaging of corneal epithelial cells [12,41]. Recently, the first toxin, acanthaporin, with pore-forming activity, cytotoxic for human neuronal cells was isolated from *Acanthamoeba*, which activation mechanism remains under investigations [12,42].

Among the indirectly contributing factors, there are amoebic and host determinants. Morphophysiological features: the amoeboid motion and spine-like acanthopodia allow protozoans to modulate binding to biological and inert surfaces. Also, changes in the overall numbers of the amoebae as well as in the proportion of trophozoites and cysts dependent on the environmental conditions are also listed as the amoebic pathogenesis determinants. The temperature tolerance, osmotolerance and growth at different pH allow the amphizoic *Acanthamoeba* to exist in different environments and simultaneously easy adapt to different human organ and tissues, including the human cornea. Moreover, it has been shown that both, clinical and environmental *Acanthamoeba* strains/isolates vary in their among the oral cavity microbiota pathogenicity. The thermal tolerance and ability to grow at high temperature are considered to be indirect markers of the pathogenicity of *Acanthamoeba* strains [12,17,18,43-45].

4. Predisposing/ risk factors sufficient to contract AK

In several studies it is underlined that the initiating of AK is a multi-factorial process, in which both host and environmental determinants are likely involved, apart connected with *Acanthamoeba* pathogenic strains [4,12].

It is considered that *Acanthamoeba* keratitis is mainly related to contact lens wear, although, *Acanthamoeba* corneal infections are also detected in persons not using contact lenses [7,12-14, 46]. After the first case of AK associated with contact lenses in Central Europe was reported from Germany, more than 85% of all incidences of the disease have been recognized in different countries in wearers of contact lenses [12,17,18,47-50].

The estimation of AK findings in several countries showed various, generally relatively low, but constantly increasing number of the cornel disease incidents during the last few decades i.e. 1.36 cases per million contact lens wears in the United States, 17 to 21 cases per million in England, 1 per 30,000 contact lens wears in France, 0.05 per 10,000 in Holland [4,12,13]. However, "it is noteworthy", as Khan [4] concluded "that variations in the incidence rate of *Acanthamoeba* keratitis do not reflect the geographical distribution of *Acanthamoeba*, and are most likely due to variations in the extended wear of soft contact lenses, varied awareness of the potential risk associated with the contact lens wear, enhanced detection, and/or local conditions that promote growth of pathogenic *Acanthamoeba* only e.g.. water hardness or salinity, or conditions that suppress growth of non-pathogenic *Acanthamoeba*." Interestingly, in Austria, women and men were affected almost equally; the highest AK incidences occurred in the 21-30-years-old patients; simultaneously, poor contact lens hygiene is indicated as the most important risk factor of AK in this country [46].

Some micro-traumas occurring earlier or appearing in connection with the use of the lenses predispose to contract AK; a human organism's susceptibility, tissue specificity, tear factors, and secretory immunoglobulin A (sIgA), important in the specific immune defense mechanism, are among other host factors influencing development of this corneal disease. Environmental conditions such as temperature, osmolarity, and pH may be important in initiating AK.

Simultaneously, the amoebae were found in contact lens and in storage cases that may be potential sources and reservoirs of the facultative parasites [12,18,47-53]. In spite of this, the incidence rate of AK in wearers of contact lenses is remarkably low in comparison with the contact lens storage cases contaminated with *Acanthamoeba*.

Additionally, it has been confirmed for various *Acanthamoeba* strains that a swimming in recreational pools while contact lenses wearing promotes the infection; it is because of some human corneal micro-defects caused by lenses and extremely high resistance of the amoebae to chlorine disinfectants [12,17, 49-53].

In persons not using contact lenses, other circumstances influence as important for contract AK [4,47]. The different *Acanthamoeba* strains are ubiquitous in natural and man-made environments thus, an exposure of the eye especially to dust, water or moist soil, as well as to any foreign particle, on which trophozoites and cyst of the amoebae can occur, is considered as an AK predisposing factor. Also, if corneal epithelial injuries appear, and also during eye surgery, circumstances promoting the infection may occur.

There have been no reports of *Acanthamoeba* keratitis being spread from one person to another.

5. When the clinician should suspect *Acanthamoeba* keratitis?

It is known, that the emerging vision-threatening AK is difficult to diagnose because clinical manifestations are similar to those observed in the course of other infectious eye diseases.

In anamnesis, in the early stage of this eye disease - patients are complaining of photophobia, excessive tearing, and reduced visual acuity; the clinical manifestations of this keratitis may also include redness and eyelid edema [13,17,50,54].

Particularly, if a presence of any foreign particles will be excluded, appearing of excruciating eye pain with intensity incommensurate with degree of corneal deterioration may suggest that *Acanthamoeba* infection develops; however, the pain not always occurs. As a rule, AK should be suspected if, in anamnesis, the contact lens wear, a history of swimming in a lake, and in recreational pools while contact lenses wearing, exposure to soil, any case of corneal trauma, surgical procedures are reported to clinician [12,18]. However, according to different reports and own experience, the amoebic etiology of the keratitis cannot be excluded in patients with above mentioned symptoms and history, previously unsuccessfully treated in ophthalmic units with antiviral, antibacterial and/or antifungal medications that delayed proper diagnosis and the suitable therapeutic management [17,50,55].

6. Differential diagnosis of AK

6.1. A tentative diagnosis of AK

The non-invasive methods are useful for the tentative diagnosis of AK, in which the slit-lamp that provides magnification from 10 to 25 times and *in vivo* confocal microscopy (Figures 2 and 3) are applied [4,12,44,50,56].

The use of a slit lamp is indicated in any acute situation that requires magnification to inspect the anterior segment of the eye. Active epithelial inflammations and hyper reflective tissues in the affected eye may be visualized by the slit lamp; a corneal ulcer and characteristic, ring-like corneal infiltration may occur in some patients. However it should be underlined that the characteristic ring infiltrate is seen in approximately 50% of AK cases.

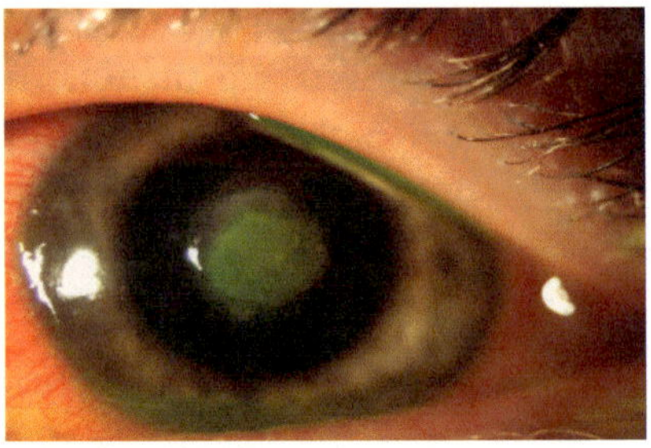

Figure 2. Slit-lamp photograph of corneal ulceration of severe *Acanthamoeba* keratitis case.

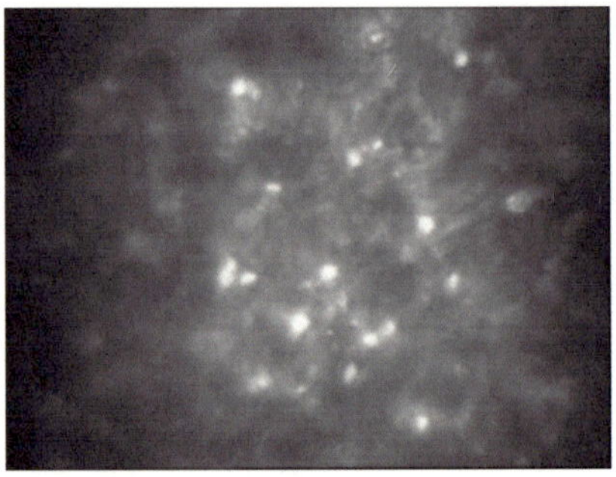

Figure 3. Hyper reflective objects - *Acanthamoeba* cysts in the affected eye with the late diagnosed severe keratitis; *in vivo* confocal microscopy; scale bar = 50μm

Different clinical presentations may occur in various causes of keratitis. However, in clinical AK practice there are nonspecific signs variable in their intensity starting with photophobia, redness, and excessive tearing that present with similar symptoms as viral, bacterial and fungal keratitis (4,7, 9-12].

In the slit lamp, corneal epithelial disease caused by *Herpes simplex* virus may be seen as dendritic keratitis or the geographic ulcer. The edges of these lesions with swollen epithelial cell stain with rose bengal while the central part stains with fluorescein [11,12,18].

Bacterial corneal infection appears typically as a one gray-white stromal infiltrate with well-demarked borders. Critical sings for fungal keratitis, e.g. *Fusarium* keratitis, are stromal gray-white or yellow-white infiltrate with a feathery border, satellite lesions surrounding the primary lesion; co-infections with fungi and bacteria can complicate the fungal keratitis [9,10,12].

In the early epithelial stage of *Acanthamoeba* keratitis, this infection can be misdiagnosed as a *Herpes simplex* keratitis because of irregular grayish lesions and pseudodendrites that are frequently observed in the epithelium. In advanced stage, AK can be mistaken as a fungal keratitis [9,11,12].

Active epithelial inflammations usually progresses from the outermost layer of the cornea -a superficial keratitis -to deeper stroma -the stromal or interstitial keratitis.

In the initial epithelial phase, typical signs of AK include epithelial or sub-epithelial infiltrates, pseudodendrites resembling these observed in *Herpes* keratitis, radial keratoneuritis (infiltrates along corneal nerves) and recurrent puncture staining of the corneal epithelium. Perineural infiltrates -a radial keratoneuritis are described as pathognomonic for the diagnosis of *Acanthamoeba* keratitis [12,18]; they are evoked by tropism of the amoebic organism for corneal nerves. Radial keratoneuritis is the reason for the extreme pain and is usually seen during the first one to four weeks of disease. Anterior stromal infiltrates are another common sing of AK. They gradually enlarge and coalesce to form a ring abscess, commonly located in the center of the cornea. Less specific signs of AK are satellite stromal infiltrates, diffuse stromal infiltrates and endothelial plaques observed in many of the patients.

Later signs of AK develop in 3-8 weeks and include a deep inflammation of the cornea consisting of a central stromal thinning and melting, anterior chamber cells and flare, hypopyon and extension of inflammation into sclera. The latter is generally reactive reaction rather than extension of infection; later in the disease course, the slowly progressive stromal opacifications and neovascularization may occur.

Etiological agents of infectious keratitis can be differing using *in vivo* confocal microscopy that is confirmed as useful tool for rapid diagnosis with high sensitivity [4,12,18,56,57].

Common findings in viral keratitis are: highly reflective, desquamating epithelial cells in superficial epithelial layer, multiple dendritic cells in basal epithelial layer, the absence of subepithelial nerve plexus, and hyperreflective keratocytes in the anterior stroma.

In bacterial keratitis, confocal micrographs typically reveal leucocytes infiltrating the corneal stroma and adherent to vessel walls. In some cases, the dendritic cells are present intrastromally; the bacteria themselves cannot be detected with the confocal microscopy.

Filamentous fungi and bacteria (e.g. *Nocardia*) can form filamentous structures that are large enough to be distinguished by confocal microscopy [57]. Another characteristics sing of filamentous fungal infection is hyphae branching, in a case of *Aspergillus* at 45° and in a case of *Fusarium* at 90°.

The examination of affected eyes by *in vivo* confocal microscopy make possible to distinguish AK from the aforementioned infectious keratitis. Lately, confocal scan features of cysts and trophozoites as well as associated corneal epithelial and stromal findings were described as criteria to specify AK in clinical diagnosis [57]. Presumable *Acanthamoeba* cysts can be visible as numerous hyper reflective, double-walled ovoid or spherical objects, 10-25μm in diameter, localized typically in deeper parts of epithelium and in anterior layers of the corneal stroma [4,18,57]. These findings should be distinguished from the well-delineated individual epithelial cell nuclei or leucocytes; the latter are larger and more regular than *Acanthamoeba* cysts. The outer wall of the cyst is more reflective than internal wall; with time, some cysts are not seen and the others become calcified. Trophozoites are also described as visible in confocal scan images, however, false results can occur because the forms are difficult to distinguish from nuclei of leukocytes and keratocytes [4,12,18]. Although confocal microscopy, if available, is non-invasive, high- sensitive tool for rapid *in vivo* diagnosis, examiners have to be familiar with morphology of *Acanthamoeba* forms. Also, differences in strain pathogenicity and viability can be taken into consideration.

It was evident also in our studies on monitoring of *in vitro* dynamics of *Acanthamoeba* strains isolated from infected eyes [17,50]; the presence of hyper reflective objects/cysts was revealed by this non-invasive *in vivo* confocal microscopy mainly for severe, late diagnosed infections with strains of which strong viability was indicated by intensive multiplying of trophozoites *in vitro* and their long survival time (42 months) in culture medium. Contrary to this, no cysts were detected by the confocal technique in material from corneal scraping if infections with weak viability strains occurred; a low amoeba number in the exponential growth phase and short (10 days) survival time of such amoeba strains were manifested *in vitro* in the culture medium. Also, no cyst was found in confocal microscopy images when mixed infections occurred, although finally the infection with *Acanthamoeba* was confirmed by laboratory methods.

Negative results of the *in vivo* confocal microscopy were reported if patients have already been pre-treated, thus the amoeba density was very low [12,50].

6.2. Why clinical manifestations are not sufficient to indicate a causative agent of keratitis

Knowledge and awareness of threat are necessary as the most important step in proper AK diagnosis as it is underlined by J. Lorenzo-Morales et al. [12].

The careful anamnesis is very important and helpful. Most of the clinical symptoms of *Acanthamoeba* keratitis are nonspecific and frequently a variability in their intensity is observed and reported from different world regions. AK is often misdiagnosed as viral infection with *Herpes simplex*, bacterial with *Pseudomonas aeruginosa* or keratitis caused by fungi of genera *Fusarium* or *Candida*; moreover, bacterial, viral, and fungal co-infections with *Acanthamoeba* may occur [2,4,46]. This is why the clinical symptoms alone, as non- pathognomonic, are not sufficient to indicate an etiological agent of human keratitis.

Undoubtedly, the non-invasive *in vivo* confocal microscopy is a valuable technique, however usefulness of it is limited if bacterial or viral keratitis occurs, thus it should be applied for the tentative diagnosis.

Also, in our several studies we analyzed serious keratitis cases regarding patients who were under suspicion of *Acanthamoeba* etiology of the infections. Although, in our hospital, finally AK was determined, there were mistakes in results of earlier diagnostics. The mixed amoebic, bacterial (*P. aeruginosa, E. faecalis*), and fungal (*Candida* sp.) infections have been revealed by us in more than 50% cases regarding persons previously unsuccessfully treated only with antibacterial and antifungal medications in other ophthalmic units [17,50].

It has been reported that *Acanthamoeba* protozoans may carry more than 20 species pathogenic for humans, among others bacteria belonging to genera *Legionella, Pseudomonas, Mycobacterium,*

Listeria and *Escherichia*, protozoa *Cryptosporidium* sp., and fungi *Cyrptococcus neoformans*. The microorganisms are able not only to survive within cells but even proliferate inside the amoebae; thus, secondary infections can occur and influence diagnostic difficulties [4,12, 18].

6.3. Laboratory evaluation

Literature data as well as results of our studies indicated that microscopic visualization of amoebae in unstained or stained slides prepared directly from corneal scraping is usefulness for AK diagnostics. Also, laboratory examinations of specimens from *in vitro* cultivated corneal isolates allow to identify directly the facultative pathogens and to verify previous misdiagnoses [4,12,46,50].

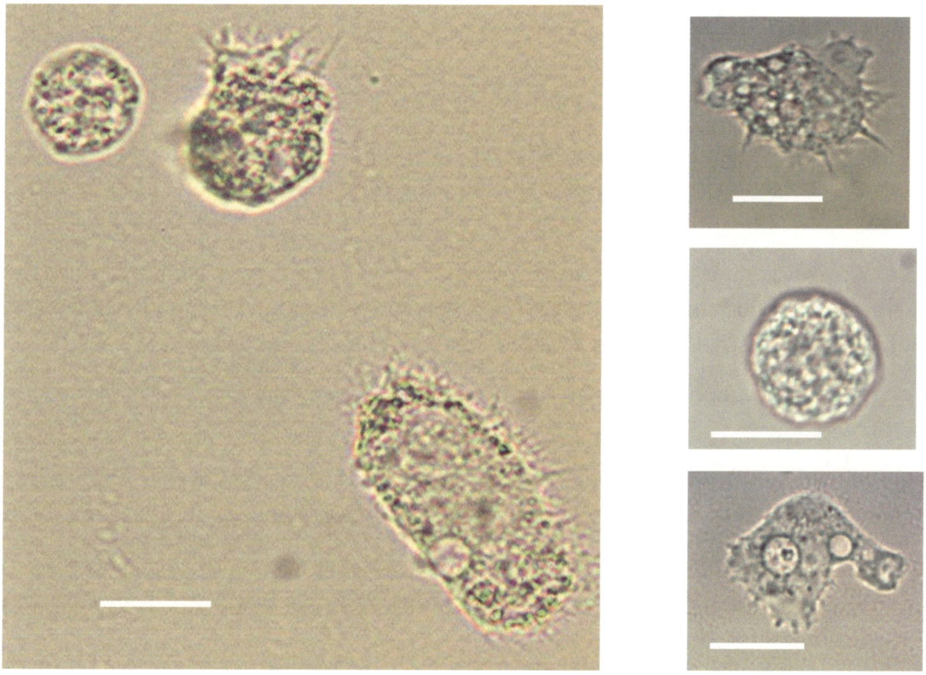

Figure 4. Live *Acanthamoeba* trophozoites and cysts in unstained preparations from corneal isolates cultured *in vitro*; light micrographs. Scale bars = 10μm

Moreover, culture methods are considered as the gold standard of diagnosis, which needs, however, collaboration between clinicians and laboratory staff and, also, the familiarization with a morphological characteristic of *Acanthamoeba* stages [12,14,18,55,58-60]. Non-nutrient (NN) agar plates seeded with Gram- negative, non-mucous bacteria: *Escherichia coli* or *Enterobacter aerogenes* are applied for isolation/growth of *Acanthamoeba* trophozoites both from environmental and clinical samples (corneal scrapings, biopsies, swabs). The incubation of the plates at 30ºC promotes a transformation of amoeba trophozoites into cysts within approximately 1 week. Also, the cultivation of amoebae in bacteria-free (axenic) conditions in a modified enriched culture medium containing antibiotics (penicillin, streptomycin) is useful for classification cysts to the morphological level.

Simultaneously, molecular methods of classification of *Acanthamoeba* isolates, with the use of sensitive PCR techniques, basing on genotype associations are distinguishing for diagnostics and for the characterization of clinical and environmental *Acanthamoeba* isolate [12,18,27,32,33,59]. In this modern approach, the species identification is based on the combination of morphological and molecular characteristics of amoebae. Additionally, our experiences gave convincing evidences of an importance of a clinical examination of the affected eyes and laboratory differentiations/identification of amoebic forms in material deriving from infected corneas.

7. Treatment options in AK

7.1. Factors complicating effective pharmacotherapy in AK

AK treatment is difficult and often unsuccessful despite of advances in pharmacotherapy. There are several factors that are listed as influencing difficulties and still not fully effective of applied therapy [12,18].

AK is often incorrect diagnosed due to nonspecific clinical symptoms; similar clinical pictures to this observed in the amoebic keratitis may give a wide range of agents e.g. viral *Herpes simplex*, bacterial -mostly *Pseudomonas aeruginosa* or fungi of *Fusarium* spp.

Additionally, mixed amoebic, fungal viral and bacterial keratitis may occur that complicate therapeutic management.

Acanthamoeba strains vary in their pathogenicity: they may be virulent, weakly virulent or non-virulent; they show different susceptibilities to chemicals and answer to pharmacotherapy.

It is also underlined that extremely high resistance of *Acanthamoeba* cysts to different chemicals, disinfectants as well as anti-microbial and anti-parasitic drugs result in disappointing therapeutic management [12,18,54,59-64].

Among the abovementioned facts, diagnostic mistakes that cause delayed in a beginning of an efficient treatment may result in a prolonged, severe course of AK and vision deterioration.

It is also emphasized that some chemicals can induce amoebic encystment that subsequently, by excystment, may lead to repeated development of trophozoites, thus an activation of the dormant cysts can lead to recurrence of the disease. It is why not only amoebicidal effects but also the cysticidal efficacy of applied therapeutics is very important [43-46].

In some research works, also in our experimental studies it has been reported that higher concentrations of drugs and some new-synthesized imidazole derivatives may be *in vitro* efficacious against *Acanthamoeba* strains and result not only in amoebostatic but also in amoebicidal effects. However, many of these chemicals cannot be applied *in vivo* in such concentrations due to their toxicity for human tissues [44-50].

http://dx.doi.org/10.5772/64848

7.2. Treatment recommended in management in AK

Currently, there are not known single-treatment methods effective against both trophozoites and cysts of *Acanthamoeba;* generally, AK is difficult to treat. *Acanthamoeba* stages differ in their susceptibility to various drugs. Trophozoite form is highly responsive to the treatment, while cysts are highly resistant as the cystic form protects the amoebic organism from unfavorable environmental factors, including drugs. The therapeutic approach recommended in AK consists of antimicrobial agent's combination [4,12,18,36].

The mainstay agents that are used as a first-line treatment for *Acanthamoeba* keratitis are diamidines (propamidine, hexamidine) and biguanides (polyhexamethylene biguanide (–PHMB), chlorhexidine), which were found to be cysticidal anti-amoebics *in vitro*. PHMB is the most preferred agent in monotherapy or in combinations with other drugs. Chlorhexidine can also be used in monotherapy, but it is much more effective in combined treatment. Propamidine is used in combination with one of biguanides, as the latter are more effective against cysts of *Acanthamoeba* [65]. Although neomycin was used widely, it is ineffective against cysts *in vitro*; thus, it is no longer used by most ophthalmologists.

However, particularly after earlier improper treatment in other centers, the combination drug therapy with the antimicrobial agents is used more or less successfully. Additionally, such factors as human organism status, a virulence of amoeba strains, phase of infection, and kind and concentration of the chemicals applied may determine variability in effects of drugs on trophozoites and cysts of several *Acanthamoeba* strains [12,16,22,45,50,64-67].

The most frequently used agents that achieve sufficient high concentrations at the site of infection and are effective against trophozoites and cysts of *Acanthamoeba* are cationic disinfectants: chlorhexidine 0.02–0.2% (200–2000 g/ml), polyhexamethylene biguanide (PHMB) 0.02–0.06% (200–600g/ml), and propamidine isethionate (Brolene 0.1%). These topical antimicrobials should be administered immediately to the infected eye one to two drops on the surface of the cornea at the first several days, every hour, minimum nine times/day, and, next, every 3h. The therapy duration is depending on clinical response. The amoebae may persist in the encysted stage for months and reactivate after therapy discontinuation. It was indicated in many earlier and current studies that a therapy continuation is very important to avoid an activation of the dormant cysts that may lead to repeated trophozoite development and thus to recurrence of the disease [4,12,13]. Some authors advise the treatment for 3- 4 months in order to preclude recurrence; however, the treatment for 6–12 months is also recommended. Nevertheless, it is reported that *Acanthamoeba* strains/cysts resistance to drug may occur, which is the main difficulty in AK treating [12,18,43,63,66]; particularly, resistance to propamidine and, also toxicity effect are observed in the course of AK. Corneal epithelial toxicity has been minimal for both chlorhexidine 0.02% and PHMB 0.02%. The greatest frequency of ocular toxicity has been reported with propamidine; the most common side effect is the superficial punctate keratopathy [65]. Pain can be relieved by topical cycloplegics (e.g. atropine 0.5-1.0%, scopolamine 0.25% t.i.d.), agents and oral non-steroidal anti-inflammatory medications (e.g. naproxen 250-500mg p.o. b.i.d.).

It should be also taken into consideration that co-infections with other microorganisms may complicate the course and treatment of the severe amoebic disease [18,49-51].

Although the low doses of topical steroids can be useful to diminish inflammation in cases of controlled infection but the use of topical corticosteroids is controversial.

Systemic corticosteroids are preferred over topical ones in cases of severe inflammation. This route of administration provides better ocular safety profile (less concentration in the cornea) but less body safety profile. However there are some suggestions that steroid use may result in increased pathogenicity of the amoebae [68].

If the topical pharmacotherapy fails, surgical interventions are needed [12,44,64,67]. Cross-linking and cryopreserved amniotic membrane graft (AMG) have been reported to be effective in AK.

The corneal transplantation can be performed for therapeutic or optical indications. Therapeutic, usually penetrating, keratoplasty is applied when the infectious process spreads to the corneal stroma, causing corneal melting and thinning despite of aggressive prolonged anti-amoebic therapy [4,12,18]. In a case of threatening or completed perforation of the cornea, the surgery must be performed urgently. Some authors recommend systemic steroids prior to surgery if concomitant limbitis or scleritis is present [69].

Sacher et al.[70] show that pretreatment of *Acanthamoeba* keratitis with intravenous pentamidine before therapeutic keratoplasty may assist with the achievement of microbiological cure, clear graft, and good visual outcome in a majority of eyes with AK.

The size of corneal graft should be minimum to excise an inflamed and necrotic tissue. Although remaining clinically healthy cornea is frequently also infected, this tissue should be saved because of the higher risk of rejection with large/decentrated grafts and because the possibility of repeat grafting should be kept in mind in the event of recurrence; a further graft represents a new food source for the organism and can be used to attract residual amoebae [69].

In a case of therapeutic keratoplasty for AK, the topical steroids in combination with anti-amoebic drugs are applied for 6-12 months following keratoplasty, to relieve pain, lessen the inflammation, and prevent graft rejection and recurrence of infection. Corneal grafts performed in the eyes with active inflammation are the high-risk transplants and they required systemic immunosuppression similar to this given in organ transplants (cyclosporine and/or mycophenolate mofetil). Apart from a poor graft survival, the postoperative glaucoma is a frequent complication.

In optical keratoplasty performed after resolution of active keratitis there is an excellent prognosis for both graft survival and visual outcome [71].

Promising clinical results were reported from amoebicidal effect of combined riboflavin and UV-A (ultraviolet light A, 365nm wavelength) exposure -corneal cross-linking (CXL) that was used for stabilization of corneal melting which can delay surgical treatment [12,72,73]. CXL has also an antimicrobial effect that is due to the effect of UV light interacting with riboflavin as the chromophore. It damages both the DNA and RNA of pathogens. Photoactivated chromophore for infectious keratitis (PACK)-CXL is an alternative to standard antibiotic therapy in treating infectious corneal disorders, and may help reduce the microbial resistance to antibiotics and avoid therapeutic keratoplasty in some cases [74].

Many chemicals and antimicrobials were examined and are still tested *in vitro* for their potential activity against different species, strains and isolates of *Acanthamoeba* [45,54,61-63,67]. Due to the toxicity of high concentrations of agents tested and a drug resistance, an optimal strategy for anti-acanthamoebic treatment is not yet defined. Further studies in this field are needed, particularly, in terms of cysticidal effects of the chemicals tested.

8. Prevention and prognosis of AK

The *Acanthamoeba* species are ubiquitous and widely distributed in natural and man-made environments. In various regions, humans were exposed frequently to the amoebae, that has been confirmed when in healthy populations specific anti- *Acanthamoeba* antibodies have been detected. For this reason, knowledge and awareness of threat are important to avoid the infection [6,12,18].

The contact lens wearers must be well educated as for the proper use and care of their lenses; do not use saline solution for lens storage, and do not to swim wearing contact lenses or use the swimming goggles. It is also very important to educate the ophthalmologist to be aware of signs and symptoms of AK and be able to early diagnose and initiate suitable treatment.

The prognosis for visual recovery with only mild residual stromal involvement is very good; in other cases, the visual prognosis is poor. Generally, a prediction depends on inflammation status at the time of diagnosis and the prompt initiation of proper treatment.

A retrospective review indicates that early diagnosis (less than 18 days) results in better final visual acuity and less likely needs keratoplasty [75]. In the early stage of infection, trophozoite forms are predominated, and the infection is confined to the superficial corneal layers. With time as the process progresses, the microorganisms enter to the deeper corneal stroma and encyst. Cysts are much more resistant to anti-protozoan drugs compared to trophozoites. Severe inflammation, scleral involvement, late diagnosis, and retardation of the therapy initialization are associated with poor clinical outcomes. In 10% of cases, there is associated scleritis. *Acanthamoeba* sclerokeratitis is associated with poor clinical outcomes [12,13,75].

9. Conclusions

Complex infective etiology and late recognition of amoebic infections were the important factors influencing diagnostic and therapeutic difficulties in AK. Laboratory examinations including *in vitro* cultivation of the isolates, acquired from corneal scrapings, allow directly to identify the facultative pathogens -the causative agents of the keratitis and to verify previous misdiagnoses. Early proper diagnosis in *Acanthamoeba* keratitis, confirmed by detection of live trophozoites in corneal scraping cultures are decisive for the treatment efficacy, particularly in contact lens wearers. The pharmacotherapy of the infectious eye disease is often unsuccessful; among others, it is if chemicals induce amoebic encystment; subsequently, an activation of the cysts can lead to repeated development of trophozoites and recurrence of the disease.

In some severe cases, keratoplasty and prolonged application of a mixture of drugs may be an appropriate option for visual rehabilitation.

Moreover, as our studies and experience show, *in vitro* monitoring of dynamics of *Acanthamoeba* strains isolated from affected eyes may be useful tool for proper diagnosis, therapeutic management and treatment prognosis.

Human infections with facultative parasitic *Acanthamoeba* strains are serious medical problem that should be taken into consideration as emerging threats of the public health worldwide.

Therefore, further educational efforts directed first of all to contact lens users are desirable for the prevention of this vision-threatening corneal disease.

Author details

Lidia Chomicz[1*], Jacek P. Szaflik[2], Marcin Padzik[1] and Justyna Izdebska[2]

*Address all correspondence to: lidia.chomicz@wum.edu.pl

1 Department of Medical Biology, Medical University of Warsaw, Warsaw, Poland

2 Department of Ophthalmology, Medical University of Warsaw, SPKSO Ophthalmic University Hospital, Warsaw, Poland

References

[1] Nagington J, Watson PG, Playfair TJ, McGill J, Jones BR, Steele ADM: Amoebic infection of the eye. Lancet. 1974;304:1537–540.

[2] Ibrahim YW, Boase DL, Cree IA: Factors affecting the epidemiology of *Acanthamoeba* keratitis. Ophthalmic Epidemiology. 2007;14:53–60.

[3] Lorenzo-Morales J, Martín-Navarro CM, López-Arencibia A, Arnalich-Montiel F, Piñero JE, Valladares B: *Acanthamoeba* keratitis: an emerging disease gathering importance worldwide? Trends in Parasitology. 2013;29(4):181–187.

[4] Khan NA: Acanthamoeba: Biology and Pathogenesis. Caister Academic Press, Norfolk, UK. 2009;290.

[5] Schroeder M, Booton GC, Hay J: Use of subgenic 18S ribosomal DNA PCR and sequencing for genus and genotype identification of *Acanthamoebae* from humans with keratitis and from sewage sludge, Journal of Clinical Microbiology. 2001;39:1903–1911.

[6] Schuster FL, Visvesvara GS: Amebic encephalitides and amebic keratitis caused by pathogenic and opportunistic free-living amebas. Current Treatment Options in Infectious Diseases. 2003;5:273–282.

[7] Marciano-Cabral F, Cabral G: *Acanthamoeba* spp. as agents of disease in humans. Clinical Microbiology Reviews. 2003;16(2):273-307.

[8] Giese MJ, Weissman BA: Contact lens associated corneal infections. Where do we go from here? Clinical & Experimental Optometry. 2002;85(3):141-148.

[9] Shah A, Sachdev A, Coggon D, Hossain P: Geographic variations in microbial keratitis: an analysis of the peer-reviewed literature. British Journal of Ophthalmology. 2011;95:762-767. doi:10.1136/bjo.2009.169607.

[10] Willcox M DP: Management and treatment of contact lens-related *Pseudomonas* keratitis. Clinical Ophthalmology. 2012: 6:919- 924. http://dx.doi.org/10.2147/OPTH.S25168.

[11] Farooq AV, Shukla D: *Herpes simplex* epithelial and stromal keratitis: an epidemiologic update. Survey of Ophthalmology. 2012;57(5):448-462. doi:10.1016/jsurvophthal.2012.01.005.

[12] Lorenzo-Morales J, Khan NA, Walochnik J: An update on *Acanthamoeba* keratitis: diagnosis, pathogenesis and treatment. Parasite. 2015;22:1-20.

[13] Trabelsi H, Dendana F, Sellami A, Sellami H, Cheikhrouhou F, Neji S, Makni F, Ayadi A: Pathogenic free-living amoebae: Epidemiology and clinical review. Pathologie Biologie. 2012;60:399–405.

[14] Khan NA: *Acanthamoeba*: biology and increasing importance in human health. FEMS Microbiology Reviews. 2006;30:564–595.

[15] Booton GC, Joslin CE, Shoff M: Genotypic identification of *Acanthamoeba* sp. isolates associated with an outbreak of *Acanthamoeba* keratitis. Cornea. 2009;28(6):673–676.

[16] Alizadeh H, Apte S, El-Agha MS: Tear IgA and serum IgG antibodies against *Acanthamoeba* in patient with *Acanthamoeba* keratitis. Cornea. 2001;20:622–627.

[17] Chomicz L, Conn DB, Padzik M, Szaflik JP, Walochnik J, Zawadzki PJ, Pawłowski W, Dybicz M: Emerging threats for human health in Poland: pathogenic isolates from drug resistant *Acanthamoeba* keratitis monitored in terms of their *in vitro* dynamics and temperature adaptability. BioMed Research International. 2015:Article ID 231285, 8pages, doi:10.1155/2015/231285.

[18] Khan NA: Acanthamoeba: Biology and Pathogenesis 2nd ed, Caister Academic Press. Norfolk, UK. 2015;295.

[19] Rodriguez-Zaragoza S, Magana-Becerra A: Prevalence of pathogenic *Acanthamoeba* (Protozoa: Amoebidae) in the atmosphere of the city of San Luis Potosi, Mexico. Toxicology & Industrial Health. 1997;13:519–526.

[20] Kilic A, Tanyuksel M, Sissons J, Jayasekera S, Khan NA: Isolation of *Acanthamoeba* isolates belonging to T2, T3, T4 and T7 genotypes from environmental samples in Ankara, Turkey. Acta Parasitologica. 2004;49(246):252.

[21] Martinez AJ, Visvesvara GS: Free-living, amphizoic and opportunistic amebas. Brain Pathology. 1997;7:583–598.

[22] Łanocha N, Kosik-Bogacka D, Maciejewska A, Sawczuk M, Wilk A, Kuźna-Grygiel W: The occurrence *Acanthamoeba* (free living amoeba) in environmental and respiratory samples in Poland. Acta Protozoologica. 2009;48(3):271–279.

[23] Nagyová V, Nagy A, Jane ček Š, Timko J: Morphological,physiological, molecular and phylogenetic characterization of new environmental isolates of *Acanthamoeba* spp. from the region of Bratislava, Slovakia. Biologia. 2010;65(1):81–91.

[24] Mahmoudi MR, Taghipour N, Eftekhar M, Haghighi A, Karanis P: Isolation of *Acanthamoeba* species in surface waters of Gilan province-north of Iran. Parasitology Research. 2012;110(1):473–477.

[25] Visvesvara GS, Moura H, Shuster FL: Pathogenic and opportunistic free-living amoebae: *Acanthamoeba* spp., *Balamuthia mandrillaris, Naegleria fowleri* and *Sappinia diploidea.* FEMS Immunology and Medical Microbiology. 2007;50:1–26.

[26] Schuster FL, Visvesvara GS: Free-living amoebae as opportunistic and non-opportunistic pathogens of humans and animals. International Journal for Parasitology. 2004a;34:1001–1027.

[27] Trabelsi H, Sellami A, Dendena F, Sellami H, Cheikh-rouhou F, Makni F, S. Ben Dhiaa'Ayadi A: Free-living amoebae (FLA): morphological and molecular identification of *Acanthamoeba* in dental unit water. Amibes libres : identification morphologique et moléculaire d'*Acanthamoeba* dans l'eau des unités dentaires. Parasite. 2010;17:67–70.

[28] Mazur T, Hadas E, Iwanicka I: The duration of the cyst stage and the viability and virulence of *Acanthamoeba* isolates. Tropical Medicine and Parasitology. 1995;46:106–108.

[29] Poussard M, Pons R: Morphologies de la paroi kystique et taxonomie du genre *Acanthamoeba* (Protozoa, Amoebida). Protistologica. 1997;13:557-610.

[30] Page FC: A New Key to Fresh Water and Soil Gymnamoebae, Freshwater Biological Association Scientific Publications, Ambleside. 1988;122.

[31] Khan NA, Jarroll EL, Paget TA: Molecular and physiological differentiation between pathogenic and nonpathogenic *Acanthamoeba,* Current Microbiology. 2002;45:197-202.

[32] Rivière D, Szczebara FM, Berjeaud JM, Frère J, Héchard Y: Development of a realtime PCR assay for quantification of *Acanthamoeba* trophozoites and cysts. Journal of Microbiological Methods. 2006; 64(1):78–83.

[33] Risler A, Coupat-Goutaland B, Pelandakis M: Genotyping and phylogenetic analysis of *Acanthamoeba* isolates associated with keratitis. Parasitology Research. 2013;112(11):3807-3816.

[34] Chappell CL, Wright JA, Coletta M, Newsome AL: Standardized method of measuring *Acanthamoeba* antibodies in sera from healthy human subjects. Clinical and Diagnostic Laboratory Immunology. 2001;8:724–730.

[35] Brindley N, Matin A, Khan NA: *Acanthamoeba castellanii*: high antibody prevalence in racially and ethnically diverse populations. Experimental Parasitology. 2009;121:254–256.

[36] Schuster FL, Visvesvara GS: Opportunistic amoebae: challenges in prophylaxis and treatment. Drug Resistance Updates. 2004b;7:41–51.

[37] Teknos TN, Poulin MD, Laruentano AM, Li KK: *Acanthamoeba* rhinosinusitis: characterization, diagnosis and treatment. American Journal of Rhinology. 2000;14:387–391.

[38] van Hamme C, Dumont M, Delos M, Lachapelle JM: Cutaneous acanthamoebiasis in a lung transplant patient. Annales de Dermatologie et de Vénéréologie. 2001;128:1237–1240.

[39] Chomicz L, Piekarczyk J, Starościak B, Fiedor P, Piekarczyk B, Szubińska D, Zawadzki PJ, Walski M: Comparative studies on the occurrence of protozoans, bacteria and fungi in the oral cavity of patients with systemic disorders. Acta Parasitologica. 2002;47:147–153.

[40] Jones B, Visvesvara GS and Robinson NM: *Acanthamoeba polyphaga* keratitis and *Acanthamoeba* uveitis associated with fatal meningoencephalitis, Transactions of the Ophthalmological Societies of the United Kingdom. 1975;95:221-232.

[41] Pellegrin JL, Ortega-Barria E, Barza M, Baum J, Pereira ME: Neuraminidase activity in *Acanthamoeba* species trophozoites and cysts. Investigative Ophthalmology and Visual Science. 1991;32:3061–3066.

[42] Michalek M, Sönnichsen FD, Wechselberger R, Dingley AJ, Hung CW, Kopp A,Wienk H, Simanski M, Herbst R, Lorenzen I, Marciano-Cabral F, Gelhaus C, Gutsmann T, Tholey A, Grötzinger J, Leippe M: Structure and function of a unique pore-forming protein from a pathogenic *Acanthamoeba*. Nature Chemical Biology. 2013;9:37–42.

[43] Aksozek A, McClellan K, Howard K: Resistance of *Acanthamoeba castellanii* cysts to physical, chemical and radiological conditions. Journal of Parasitology. 2002;88:621-623.

[44] Szaflik JP, Padzik M, Chomicz L, Oledzka G, Izdebska J: Usefulness of *in vitro* diagnostics in difficult incidences of *Acanthamoeba* keratitis requiring pharmacotherapy and surgical management. Okulistyka. 2012;3:28–32.

[45] Chomicz L, Padzik M, Graczyk Z, Starociak B, Graczyk T., Naprawska A, Olędzka G, Szostakowska B: *Acanthamoeba castellanii*: *in vitro* effects of selected biological, physical and chemical factors. Experimental Parasitology. 2010;126,103–105.

[46] Walochnik J, Scheikl U, Haller-Schober EM: Twenty years of *Acanthamoeba* diagnostics in Austria. Journal of Eukaryotic Microbiology. 2015;62(1),3–11.

[47] Padzik M, Chomicz L, Szaflik JP, Chruscikowska A, Perkowski K, Szaflik J: *In vitro* effects of selected contact lens care solutions on *Acanthamoeba castellanii* strains in Poland. Experimental Parasitology. 2014;145:98–101.

[48] Witschel H, Sundmacher R, Seitz HM: Amebic keratitis: clinico-histopathologic case report. Klinische Monatsblatter fur Augenheilkunde: 1984;185:46–49.

[49] Moore MB, McCulley JB, Luckenbach M: *Acanthamoeba* keratitis associated with soft contact lenses. American Journal of Ophthalmology. 1985;100:396–403.

[50] Chomicz L, Padzik M, Szaflik JP, Nahorski WL, Kryczka T, Szaflik J: Monitoring of *in vitro* dynamics of *Acanthamoeba* strains isolated from infected eyes as a useful tool in keratitis management. Experimental Parasitology. 2014;145:73-77.

[51] Larkin DFP, Kilvington S, Easty L: Contamination of contact lens storage cases by *Acanthamoeba* and bacteria. British Journal of Ophthalmology. 1990;74:133–135.

[52] Hiti K, Walochnik J, Haller-Schober EM, Faschinger C, Aspock H: Viability of *Acanthamoeba* after exposure to a multipurpose disinfecting contact lens solution and two hydrogen peroxide systems. British Journal of Ophthalmology. 2002;86:144–146.

[53] Hiti K, Walochnik J, Faschinger C, Haller-Schober EM, Aspock H: One- and two-step hydrogen peroxide contact lens disinfection solutions against *Acanthamoeba*: how effective are they? Eye. 2005;19:1301–1305.

[54] Chomicz L, Zebrowska J, Piekarczyk J, Starosciak B, Myjak P, Walski M, Kazimierczuk Z: *In vitro* studies on susceptibility of *Acanthamoeba castellanii* to selected chemical agents. Acta Parasitologica. 2005;50:25–31.

[55] da Rocha-Azevedo B, Tanowitz HB, Marciano-Cabral F: Diagnosis of infections caused by pathogenic free-living amoebae. Hindawi Publishing Corporation. Interdisciplinary Perspectives on Infectious Diseases. 2009:1–14. ID 251406.

[56] Winchester K, Mathers WD, Sutphin JE, Daley TE: Diagnosis of *Acanthamoeba* keratitis *in vivo* with confocal microscopy. Cornea. 1995;14(1):10-17.

[57] Rezaei Kanavi M, Naghshgar N, Javadi MA, Sadat Hashemi M: Various confocal scan features of cysts and trophozoites in cases with *Acanthamoeba* keratitis. European Journal of Ophthalmology. 2012; 22:46-50.

[58] Schuster FL: Cultivation of pathogenic and opportunistic free-living amebas. Clinical Microbiology Reviews. 2002;15(3):342–354.

[59] Lass A, Szostakowska B, Idzińska A, Chomicz L: The first genotype determination of *Acanthamoeba* potential threat to human health, isolated from natural water reservoirs in Poland. Parasitology Research. 2014;113(7):2693-2699.

[60] Walochnik J, Obwaller A, Aspock H: Correlations between morphological, molecular biological, and physiological characteristics in clinical and nonclinical isolates of *Acanthamoeba* spp. Applied and Environmental Microbiology. 2000;66:4408–4413.

[61] Lloyd D, Turner NA, Khunkitti W, Hann AC, Furr JR, Russell AD: Encystation in *Acanthamoeba castellanii*: development of biocide resistance. Journal of Eukaryotic Microbiology. 2001;48:11–16.

[62] Kopanska K, Najda A, Zebrowska J, Chomicz L, Piekarczyk J, Myjak P, Bretner M: Synthesis and activity of 1H-benzimidazole and 1H-benzotriazole derivatives as inhibitors of *Acanthamoeba castellanii.* Bioorganic & Medicinal Chemistry. 2004;12:2617-2624.

[63] Turner NA, Russell AD, Furr JR, Lloyd D: Emergence of resistance to biocides during differentiation of *A. castellanii.* Journal of Antimicrobial Chemotherapy. 2000;46:27–34.

[64] Chomicz L, Szaflik JP, Padzik M, Oledzka G, Iwanczyk B, Szaflik J: Anti-amoebic chemotherapeutics and surgical procedures in *Acanthamoeba* keratitis difficult to diagnose. In: Proceedings of 47th Congress of the European Society for Surgical Research, 6-9 June, 2012, Lille, France. Medimond International Proceedings. 2012;55–57.

[65] Yolton DP, Haesaert SP: Anti-infective drugs. Bartlett JD, Jaanus SD. Clinical Ocular Pharmacology. 5th ed. Elsevier. Butterworth Heinemann. 2008

[66] Ficker L, Seal D, Warhurst D, Wright P: *Acanthamoeba* keratitis- resistance to medical therapy. Eye. 1990;4:835–838.

[67] Chomicz L, Padzik M, Izdebska J, Baltaza W, Wroczynski P, Szaflik JP: *In vitro* activity of toyocamycin and novel thioinozine derivative as potential drugs against amphizoic amoebae -the causative agents of *Acanthamoeba* keratitis. The International Symposium on Ocular Pharmacology and Therapeutics. 12th ISOPT Clinical, Berlin, Germany, July 9-12. Session: Inflammation and Infection, Abstracts. 2015;732.

[68] Robaei D, Carnt N, Minassian DC, Dart JK: The impact of topical corticosteroid use before diagnosis on the outcome of *Acanthamoeba* keratitis. Ophthalmology. 2014;121(7):1383–1388.

[69] Graffi S, Peretz A, Jabaly H Naftali M: *Acanthamoeba* Keratitis. Israel Medical Association Journal. 2013; 15:182–185.

[70] Sacher BA, Wagoner MD, Goins KM, Sutphin JE, Greiner MA, Kitzmann AS: Treatment of *Acanthamoeba* keratitis with intravenous pentamidine before therapeutic keratoplasty. Cornea. 2015;34(1):49-53.

[71] Kitzmann AS, Goins KM, Sutphin JE, Wagoner MD: Keratoplasty for treatment of *Acanthamoeba* keratitis. Ophthalmology. 2009;116(5):864-869. doi:10.1016/j.ophtha.2008.12.029.

[72] Garduño-Vieyra L, González-Sánchez CR, Hernández-Da Mota SE: Ultraviolet-A light and riboflavin therapy for *Acanthamoeba* keratitis: a case report. Case Reports in Ophthalmology. 2011;2(2):291–295.

[73] Khan YA, Kashiwabuchi RT, Martins SA, Castro-Combs JM, Kalyani S, Stanley P, Flikier D, Behrens A: Riboflavin and ultraviolet light a therapy as an adjuvant treatment for medically refractive *Acanthamoeba* keratitis: report of 3 cases. Ophthalmology. 2011;118(2),324–331.

[74] Tabibian D, Richoz O, Hafezi F: PACK-CXL: Corneal cross-linking for treatment of infectious keratitis. Journal Ophthalmic and Vision Research. 2015;10(1):77-80.

[75] Claerhout I, Goegebuer A, Van Den Broecke C., Kestelyn P:Delay in diagnosis and outcome of *Acanthamoeba* keratitis. Graefes Archive for Clinical and Experimental Ophthalmology. 2004;242(8):648-653.

Chapter 5

Eye Coinfections

Carlos Alberto Pantoja-Meléndez, Victor M. Bautista-de Lucio, Mariana Ortiz-Casas, Jonathan Quevedo-Martínez and Herlinda Mejía-López

Additional information is available at the end of the chapter

http://dx.doi.org/10.5772/64702

Abstract

Ocular infections are an *ophthalmologic* emergency that threatens the eye's integrity, which may result in a poor visual outcome; hence, it requires prompt treatment. The most common microorganisms involved in eye infection are the bacteria, followed by virus and fungi; however the prevalence depends on the geographic location. It is essential to know The etiologic agent of the ocular infection ocular infections and their antibiotic sensitivity because the geographical situation and the urbanization level of the studied population will determine their prevalence. Recently have been described eye coinfections, where at least two microorganisms can infect at the same time and the same anatomic site. Several coinfections have been published, bacteria-bacteria, bacteria-fungus, bacteria-virus, fungus-yeast, fungus-virus, parasite-bacteria, etc. Eye coinfections represent a particular challenge for the ophthalmologists; coinfections are difficult to diagnose because often the clinical characteristic is atypical and mimics different clinical pictures. In addition, eye coinfections respond poorly to antibiotics and usually present an aggressive clinical course. In these circumstances, it is common for patients to receive multiple treatments when they should be receiving a specific treatment. Several risk factors are important to develop coinfections, e.g., trauma, dry eye, use of contact lenses, and comorbidities (diabetes and immunosuppression). Coinfections have been described in keratitis, conjunctivitis, and endophthalmitis. The study of polymicrobial biofilms has been increasing, and in the medical area, the role played by biofilms in confections has been associated with virulence factors; hence, biofilm formation is also considered a determinant virulence factor for pathogenesis in the host. Coinfection diagnosis is an important topic in order to obtain a specific and timely diagnosis. Microbiological and molecular approaches are proposed to identify etiological agents. Delay in diagnosis affects the sensitivity to specific treatments and the evolution of infection. Treatment and prognosis are supported by a specific diagnosis.

Keywords: Coinfection, polyinfections, biofilm

1. Introduction

An infected eye is one of the major causes of corneal blindness after cataract in developing countries [1]. This is mainly induced by bacteria, fungi, yeast, and parasites. However, an increasing number of coinfections, which involve the presence of two or more pathogens, in the same place at the same time, affecting one or both eyes, are being reported. Comparing the single-microorganism infections, in which theoretically there is no competition, the coinfections have been proven to have more mechanisms competing against the host resources. This competition is the main factor influencing the clinical course and evolution of the infection [2].

Eye coinfections represent a particular challenge for ophthalmologists; coinfections are difficult to diagnose because often the clinical picture is atypical and mimics different clinical pictures. In addition, eye coinfections respond poorly to antibiotics and usually present a slow clinical course. In these circumstances, it is common for patients to receive multiple treatments when they should be receiving a specific treatment; this can cause a refractory infection and need for surgical treatments.

Although eye infections are common in immunocompetent patients, coinfection can compromise the immune system of the host [3, 4]. Therefore, the strategies used by each microorganism to survive against different treatments and the self-host immune response have important implications for the diagnosis and prognosis of the infection [5].

This chapter provides a systematic review of the frequency and epidemiological characteristics, with reports of the most common clinical entities, produced by coinfection in the eye.

2. Epidemiological characteristics

2.1. Epidemiological significance

Ocular infectious processes are among the clinical entities that are relevant to the epidemiology. The high incidence of infections in patient care institutions has resulted in high-quality infection control processes and monitoring of various entities of epidemiological relevancy. For example, viral conjunctivitis primarily represents a challenge for management and prevention. Thus, it is common for diseases such as hemorrhagic conjunctivitis and follicular conjunctivitis to be part of the epidemiological surveillance.

The difficulty of the epidemiological surveillance of ophthalmic diseases lies in the limitation of performing a specific etiologic diagnosis of infection, since in practice ophthalmic infections are treated empirically based on the clinical picture and the physician's experience. Ophthalmologists and laboratory staff should not forget that care of patients with endophthalmitis is usually performed at the first level of care, where the general practice is responsible for the greatest amount of attention to this disease. Thus, control programs for conditions such as trachoma are necessary to prevent them from reemerging and being attentive and vigilant regarding emerging diseases.

http://dx.doi.org/10.5772/64702

Within emerging diseases, changes are observed in response to treatment but more important in the modification to the incidence and prevalence to disease. Reports of bacterial strain resistant to antibiotics and changes in the behavior expected of diseases are increasing. Therefore, new mechanisms of resistance of microorganisms, comorbidity states in individuals, new mechanisms of transmission, etc., that explain what changes in the conditions have occurred are sought. One explanation is the presence of more than one causal agent of infectious disease, coinfections.

The mechanisms developed by various microorganisms when present concurrently can alter significantly the clinical presentation, diagnosis, and treatment.

Coinfections resemble clinical pictures presented by other clinical entities and have an adverse effect, as the usual outcome is the use of multi-treatment that fails, causing refractory management and in many cases ending in loss of vision or surgical interventions. This reveals the importance of presenting cases of coinfections of the eye.

Although eye coinfections are not the subject of epidemiological surveillance, they are not as rare as previously thought and can represent 3.88 % of endophthalmitis cases, for example, and more than 50 % in some series of patients with conjunctivitis reported in the literature [6, 7].

3. Agents

Associated microorganisms may occur in different combinations. This association is predominantly bacteria-bacteria and to a lesser extent bacteria-fungus and bacteria-virus.

Acanthamoeba spp. and *Pseudomonas* spp. are associated because of their high resistance to empirical antibiotics and ulceration, which occurs primarily in association with *Acanthamoeba* spp., which is associated with *Legionella* spp., *Streptococcus* spp., herpes virus, *Moraxella* spp., *Candida* spp., etc.

Several viruses, bacteria, or fungi cause eye infections, but the pathogenic agent is modified extensively at presentation as a coinfection especially when the bacterium is coinfecting with different bacteria or a virus. In the case of fungi, when they are present with bacteria, only small changes are observed [3]. The clinical spectrum of keratitis can change when there is a coinfection between bacteria and *Candida* spp., mainly occurs; however, when endophthalmitis involves coinfection of a fungus and Gram-negative bacteria, the result is more unfavorable [6].

4. Risk factors

The core components of the presentation of coinfections are risk factors. However, studies have not shown high causality for association. Coinfections have been diagnosed in patients with no reports of comorbidities (diabetes, immunosuppressive processes, etc.) although coinfections can occur in patients with human immunodeficiency virus (HIV); however, this risk factor was not significant in the patients reported.

One risk factor for coinfection of fungus and bacteria is trauma. Dry eye also seems to be a risk factor.

The most frequently reported risk factor is the use of contact lenses, especially soft lenses. Coinfection with *Acanthamoeba* spp. *and Pseudomonas* spp. has been reported in contact lens-associated keratitis. Poor response to treatment has been observed in young people with greater frequency in women.

5. Challenges

The most important challenge in the emergence of this clinical entity is the identification of a new form of presentation of eye infections. The standard method of causality associates the disease with a single causative agent. However, in this new scenario, more than one causal agent is observed. The new entity must be monitored and addressed as a new disease, which requires a new diagnostic approach, prognosis, and treatment.

6. Keratitis due to coinfections

6.1. Bacteria and fungus

Bacteria and fungus represent the most frequent type of coinfection in the eye (Table 1]. The main microorganisms that produce coinfections are bacteria, such as *Staphylococcus* spp., *Streptococcus* spp., *Pseudomonas* spp., *Haemophilus* spp., *Klebsiella* spp., *Bacillus* spp., and *Corynebacterium* spp. The fungi genera microorganisms include *Aspergillus* spp., *Fusarium* spp., *Curvularia* spp., *Cladosporium* spp., *Bipolaris* spp., *Alternaria* spp., and the yeast *Candida* spp. Most of these microorganisms are normal microbiota in the conjunctival sac or the lids [8]. Their presence depends on the geographic area. However, bacteria and fungus coinfections that have been reported more frequently in a large series of cases are the genera *Staphylococcus* spp. with *Aspergillus* spp. or *Fusarium* spp., [3, 9, 10, 11, 12, 13].

Organisms	Study type	Infection caused	Reference
Bacteria and fungus	Transversal	Keratitis	Gopinathan *et. al.* 2009
	Transversal	Keratitis	Basak *et. al.* 2005
	Transversal	Keratitis	Pate *et. al.* 2006
	Transversal	Keratitis	Bharathi *et. al.* 2002
Bacteria and bacteria	Transversal	Keratitis	Fröhlich *et. al.* 1999
	Transversal	Keratitis	Yeh *et. al.* 2006
	Case	Keratitis	Jones 1981

http://dx.doi.org/10.5772/64702

Organisms	Study type	Infection caused	Reference
Bacteria and yeast	Case	Keratitis	Kim *et. al.* 2006
Filamentous fungus and yeast	Case	Keratitis	Qui *et. al.* 2013
Filamentous fungus and filamentous fungus	Case	Keratitis	Hayashi *et. al.* 2014
Acanthamoeba and bacteria	Transversal	Keratitis	Tu *et. al.* 2009
	Case	Keratitis	Hong *et. al.* 2014
	Case	Keratitis	Dini *et. al.* 2000
	Transversal	Keratitis	Iovieno *et. al.* 2010
	Case	Keratitis	Lone *et. al.* 2009
Acanthamoeba and fungus	Transversal	Keratitis	Froumis *et. al.* 2008
	Case	Keratitis	Gupta *et. al.* 2011
	Case	Keratitis	Slade *et. al.* 2008
Virus and bacteria	Case	Conjunctivitis	Mellman-Rubin *et. al.* 1995
	Case	Conjunctivitis	Tappe *et. al.* 2013
Bacteria and bacteria	Transversal	Conjunctivitis	Iwalokun *et. al.* 2011
Bacteria and bacteria	Transversal	Endophthalmitis	Gharamah *et. al.* 2012
	Transversal	Endophthalmitis	Jindal *et. al.* 3013
	Transversal	Endophthalmitis	Gupta *et. al.* 2002
Bacteria and fungus	Transversal	Endophthalmitis	Long *et. al.* 2014
	Transversal	Endophthalmitis	Gupta *et. al.* 2003
HIV and herpes	Transversal	Retinal necrosis syndrome	Liesegang 2001
HIV and cytomegalovirus	Transversal	Retinitis	Faber *et. al.* 1992
HIV, Epstein-Barr, and cytomegalovirus	Transversal	Retinitis	Freigassner *et. al.* 2002
HIV, cytomegalovirus, and herpes	Case	Retinitis	Skolnik *et. al.* 1989
HIV and several microorganisms (including *Acanthamoeba*)	Case	Keratitis	Tandon *et. al.* 2003
HIV and *Treponema pallidum*	Case	Severe bilateral retinal vasculitis	Albini *et. al.* 2011
Virus and worm	Case	Perilimbal and conjunctival infection and HZV lesson	Seo *et. al.* 2014

Table 1. Main reports of human eye coinfections.

Bacterial and fungal keratitis often is not clinically distinguishable from monomicrobial infections, because they override the pathognomonic picture typical of bacterial or fungal keratitis [14]. Because of the difficulty of clinical diagnosis, other factors are added; many patients use traditional medicine (with the risk of adding other microorganisms to the infection) or initiate topical medication without a medical prescription. These therapeutic interventions delay the specific treatment, and the prognosis of infection is poor [14].

Bacteria and fungus coinfection can be incidental in the first instance. However, this condition favors the development in the participating pathogens of adaptive mechanisms that strengthen their protection versus the immune system host or the antimicrobial drug. This phenomenon is explained by the ability of fungi and bacteria to form biofilms. Studies recently showed that 99 % of microorganisms can form biofilms; only 10 % live as planktonic cells (unicellular cells) [15, 16, 17].

The characteristic that best distinguishes chronic infections from acute infections is the response to treatment with antibiotics. While acute infections can be removed after a short treatment with antibiotics, the biofilm in keratitis coinfections normally fails to be completely eliminated, produces recurrent episodes, and often must be solved with keratoplasty. The etiologic agents form biofilms that can be up to 1,000 times more resistant to antibiotics [17, 18, 19]. The issue of biofilms will be fully explained in the following section.

7. Bacteria and bacteria

Several reports in the literature have described this coinfection. Fröhlich *et. al.* studied patients with and without clinical history of contact lens use and showed that 51 of the 275 samples (18.5 %) from patients with bacteria keratitis were coinfections. The most common pathogens isolated were *Staphylococcus epidermidis* (44 %), *Staphylococcus aureus* (18 %), *Streptococcus* spp. (10 %), *Propionibacterium acnes* (7 %), and *Pseudomonas aeruginosa* (6 %) [20]. Yeh *et. al.* presented a study of 307 samples, of which 21 % were keratitis bacteria-bacteria coinfections with similar bacterial genera [21]. Jones reported coinfections between *Streptococcus pneumoniae* with *Corynebacterium* spp. or *Staphylococcus epidermidis* and isolated three microorganisms from one case, *Staphylococcus aureus* and *Streptococcus pneumoniae, Corynebacterium* spp., and *Micrococcus* spp., and, finally, *Streptococcus equinus* and *Haemophilus influenzae* from another patient.

8. Bacteria and yeast

Coinfections that involve *Candida* spp. or a filamentous fungus are usually difficult to treat, and the prognosis is poor. A coinfection of *Stenotrophomonas maltophilia* (Gram (-) bacteria) and a yeast has been documented. The corneal injury presented as an ulcer that quickly progressed despite treatment with proven sensitivity. The case was treated with penetrating keratoplasty [22].

9. Filamentous fungi and yeast

In a case with clinically distinguishable corneal infiltrates, *Exserohilum mcginnisii* and *Candida parapsilosis*, an unusual coinfection, were isolated. The infection showed torpid evolution with severe damage in the visual area [23]. Katragkou *et. al.* conducted a review that showed *Exserohilum* spp. produces a wide spectrum of diseases, including atopic, cutaneous, subcutaneous, systemic, and corneal infections; the most common factor was immunocompromised status [24]. In addition, *Candida* spp. is an opportunistic pathogen that affects immunocompromised and immunocompetent patients. This genus generates biofilms responsible for resistance to a wide range of antifungal drugs and often affects the cornea [25, 26]. *Exserohilum* spp. and *Candida* spp. can acquire a filamentous form that invades the stroma or produces endophthalmitis and has the capability of assembling biofilms.

10. Filamentous fungus and filamentous fungus

A case of sclerokeratitis produced by *Scedosporium apiospermum* and *Aspergillus cibarius* was recently reported. The case, which was characterized by insidious keratitis and liquefied sclera, was successfully treated with topical and systemic antifungal drugs [27].

11. *Acanthamoeba* spp. and coinfections

Acanthamoeba spp., a protozoon, is a free-living amoeba that can live in diverse environments. It has been isolated from soil, water for domestic use, salt or freshwater sewage, estuaries, hot springs, and swimming pools, among others, which highlight the microorganism's ability to live in extreme heat and pH conditions. Schuster and Visvesvara described *Acanthamoeba* spp. producing keratitis as non-opportunistic and thus occur in immunocompetent humans [28]. Galarza *et. al.*, described this amoeba as *amphizoic* due to its ability to live in the environment and parasitize humans [29].

The life cycle of *Acanthamoeba* spp. includes two stages: the cyst, a form of resistance to adverse environmental conditions, and the trophozoite, the amoeboid free-living stage. Due to the organism's phagocytic condition, *Acanthamoeba* spp. can feed of bacteria, algae, yeast, fungi, etc [30]; but some of these microorganisms have developed mechanisms to avoid intracellular death and take advantage of the amoeba (endosymbiosis). These circumstances make *Acanthamoeba* spp. a vector of almost any type of microorganism; Barket *et. al.*, in studies of the host-parasite relationship, called it a "Trojan horse" [31, 32].

12. *Acanthamoeba* and bacteria

The association of *Acanthamoeba* spp. with other microorganisms is most significant from the ophthalmological point of view. This species can generate corneal injuries that remain for months or years and are difficult to treat with diamine and biguanide drugs in developing countries (chlorhexidine and polyhexamethylene biguanide, respectively) [33].

Some of the bacteria mechanisms within *Acanthamoeba* spp. have been described. Scheid *et. al.*, using an *in vitro* model with electronic microscopy, showed the cycle of a coccoid-like organism in the free-living amoebae *Vannella* spp. The coccoid microorganism is a phagocyte and is transported by phagocytic vacuoles through the cytosol until reaching the amoeba nucleus where the microorganism proliferates and is released by rupture of the host membrane. In the beginning of the life cycle, coccoid microorganisms are phagocytes for other amoeba [34]. In addition, endosymbiont bacteria can replicate only into the amoeba cytosol, can break the cells, and can be ingested by neighboring amoeba [35]. However, the intrusion of bacteria into *Acanthamoeba polyphaga* has consequences for both microorganisms. A protein bellows the amoeba that adheres to the surface of *Legionella pneumophila*. The authors discussed the possibility that the liberation of the bacteria from the amoeba integrates amoeba antigens in its membrane. However, *Pseudomonas aeruginosa* and its liberated products kill *Acanthamoeba* spp. [30, 32, 36]. Another study showed that endosymbiont bacteria favor the growth of different species of *Acanthamoeba*, and all microorganisms isolated from contact lens care solutions contained numerous trophozoites [37].

Acanthamoeba spp. by itself causes severe inflammation in the cornea. Aggressive keratolysis or sclerokeratitis is a common complication. The most frequently reported symptoms are pain, photophobia, and tearing [38]. The association of *Acanthamoeba* spp. with bacteria or a fungus presents a coinfection that can mimic bacterial, fungal, or herpetic keratitis, which can delay the time to diagnosis and increase the pathogenicity of the *Acanthamoeba* spp. infection.

Several molecular methods and electronic microscopy have facilitated the observation of bacteria within *Acanthamoeba*, including *Pseudomonas aeruginosa*, *Listeria monocytogenes*, *Mycobacterium* spp., *Escherichia coli*, *Legionella pneumophila*, *Chlamydia* spp., and *Aeromonas* spp. They are also capable of producing keratitis themselves [30, 32, 39, 40, 41]. In addition, there are many reports in the literature of cases of *Acanthamoeba* and bacteria coinfection isolated from patients with or without contact lens-associated keratitis [39, 42, 43, 44].

13. *Acanthamoeba* and fungi

This type of coinfection is uncommon. Similar to bacteria, fungi have a complex relationship with *Acanthamoeba* spp. and generate lesions that can be confused with bacterial or herpetic keratitis; the prognosis is discouraging. In all cases reported, penetrating keratoplasty was performed. These coinfections require immediate and aggressive treatment with antifungal and antiamoebic drugs [45, 46, 47, 48, 49].

14. Conjunctivitis due to coinfection

Conjunctivitis is the most common eye infection in the world. Usually, the normal microbiota in the conjunctiva participates in infectious diseases of the ocular surface, and it has been reported that diversity in the conjunctival microbiota varies depending on geographic region or occupational activity [50, 51, 52, 53]. Moreover, the pathogenesis of infectious conjunctivitis depends on the circumstances and intrinsic mechanisms to the microorganism and the host.

Although there are high diversity of microorganisms on the conjunctiva, few coinfections have been reported. This lack of reports could be due to confusing clinical manifestations or the low sensitivity of the methods used or simply because two or more microorganisms are not usually searched in an infection.

In a patient with conjunctivitis, an uncommon relationship between an adenovirus and *Chlamydia* spp. was reported. The study showed three patients positive for *Chlamydia* spp. in a sample of 100 patients with adenoviral conjunctivitis, using polymerase chain reaction (PCR) [54, 55]. Another report showed the presence of adenovirus type 53 with a multiple resistant strain of *Neisseria gonorrhoeae* in a patient with severe bilateral conjunctivitis.

Iwalokun *et. al.*, presented interesting results in a study conducted in Lagos, Nigeria. They analyzed 83 samples from patients with conjunctivitis and isolated 155 bacteria from the samples; the resistance patterns and the plasmid profile were evaluated. The authors found coinfections of two, three, or more pathogens (51.8 % and 18.1 %, respectively) and were able to identify three infection patterns that were significantly different [7]. This work emphasizes the possibility that multiple microorganisms can cause conjunctivitis.

15. Endophthalmitis due to coinfection

Endophthalmitis is an inflammatory intraocular reaction and is the most important complication for an ophthalmologist following surgery, trauma, and between others. The common presentation of the clinical picture is characterized by pain and decreased vision. As previously discussed in the section on keratitis due to bacteria and fungus coinfections, endophthalmitis due to coinfection can be confused with single bacterial or fungal infections. Thus, to facilitate successful interventions, the microorganisms responsible must be identified and antimicrobial sensitivity examined. Studies of several large series have shown the frequency of endophthalmitis due to bacteria and fungus and bacteria and bacteria coinfections.

Depending on patients' geographic region, consecutive case studies have found various incidence rates for this coinfection ranging from 2.4 % to 50 % [56, 57, 58, 59].

The most commonly isolated pathogens are Gram-positive cocci bacteria with filamentous fungi [60, 61]. However, Gram-negative or Gram-positive bacilli related to fungi are also responsible for endophthalmitis [60, 61, 62].

16. Coinfections in immunocompromised patients

The outcome of coinfection is the result of diverse interactions involving the host and the parasite's genetic background and the environment. In these infections, few reports have explained the immune mechanisms implicated, because there is considerable variability in each combination of microorganisms that produces an infection.

The immunological mechanisms that occur in the eye are similar to the rest of the immune system. However, there is more regulation in the silencing response in order to prevent damage from infection and inflammation, and immune mechanisms preserve the functionality of the cornea [63].

In the following, studies that investigated the most common corneal coinfections are reviewed. These reports show the critical role of pathogens and the pathogenesis generated by the host immune response.

Vernal conjunctivitis is an example of how the immune phenotype affects the response to the infection. Patients with vernal keratoconjunctivitis have a family history of atopic diseases such as allergic rhinitis, asthma, and eczema [64]. A theory suggests that patients with a history of atopy are susceptible to intracellular infections because they have a Th2 immune phenotype [65, 66]. Kerr and Stern showed a polymicrobial infection in two patients with vernal keratoconjunctivitis and corneal ulcers [67].

Although regulation of the immune response in the eye is controlled locally, in immunocompromised patients with human immunodeficiency virus (HIV), it is evident that the privilege is broken by the depletion of T CD4+ cells, and infections can occur. In addition, several pathogens can remain latent (herpes virus, bacteria, fungi, parasites). The clinical manifestation produced by the herpes virus can be conjunctivitis, blepharitis, intraocular inflammation, retinitis, or keratitis [68]. In particular, herpes simplex virus types 1 and 2 (HSV-1 and HSV-2] infect 50 % to 90 % of the population infected with HIV, causing ocular herpes and genital orofacial herpes in different geographic regions [69]. Herpetic retinitis has a high incidence; however, few cases have been reported. Faber *et. al.*, studied eyes from 25 cases with AIDS with an immunohistochemical test. *Cytomegalovirus* was found in 60 % of the cases and was related to retinitis, while in another case series, 36.64 % of 131 patients were diagnosed with *Cytomegalovirus* retinitis [70, 71]. Freigassner *et. al.*, documented a case with the Epstein-Barr virus and *Cytomegalovirus* in a patient with AIDS [72]. Other studies showed *Cytomegalovirus* or herpes in isolated cases [73, 74, 75].

Opportunistic microorganisms such as *Toxoplasma* spp., herpes zoster virus (HZV), and *Pneumocystis* spp., participates the least in coinfections.

17. Coinfections produced by strange conjunction of pathogens

Burkholderia ambifaria, Enterococcus, and *Staphylococcus aureus* were found in a patient with herpetic stromal keratitis. *Burkholderia ambifaria* is a Proteobacteria, which comprises strains with a virulence potential toward immunocompromised patients [76]. In a report on keratitis, *Acanthamoeba* spp., *Fusarium solani,* and Gram-negative cocci were identified in a patient who had unprotected sexual contact with multiple commercial sex workers [77].

http://dx.doi.org/10.5772/64702

18. Pharmacodynamics of antimicrobials used in eye coinfections

There is little information about the pharmacodynamics of antimicrobials used for coinfections of the human eye. The activity of antimicrobial drugs against yeast, bacteria, and fungi has been evaluated with a standardized microdilution assay in a culture medium [78]. The lowest concentration of an antimicrobial that completely inhibits the growth of any microorganism is known as the minimal inhibitory concentration (MIC), which can be used to determine the sensitivity or resistance.

Based on MICs with microdilutions and the growth radial technique on solid medium using Potato Dextrose Agar (PDA) dishes (using the percent mycelial inhibition) [79], our group reported that *S. aureus* cocultured with *F. solani* or *A. fumigatus* (all isolated from patients) significantly inhibited fungal growth (66.5 % and 55.6 %, respectively). gatifloxacin and moxifloxacin in the cocultures eliminated the bacterial effect on both growth fungi ($p<0.001$). amphotericin B, natamycin, and itraconazole inhibited fungal growth partially or completely, depending on the fungus. In contrast, the effect of amphotericin B or natamycin in the presence of quinolones significantly favored the growth of fungi; this effect was more evident in *F. solani* [80].

Nevertheless, the MIC does not reflect physiological concentrations of drugs because *in vivo* drug concentrations may vary due to many factors such as absorption, metabolism, half-life, elimination, etc. [81, 82, 83]. In addition, in treatments with prophylactic and therapeutic purposes for confections, fortified or coadministered agents are used that may affect the efficacy of the other agent [84, 85].

Attempts to understand the magnitude and type of interactions between drugs have enabled the development in isobolographic analysis of the "gold standard" for drug interactions, which define the interactions as follows: *Additive effect*: The combined effect of two drugs (A and B) equals the sum of the equivalent doses (depending on the relative potency of each drug). *Synergism*: The effect of A and B is greater than that of the two separate drugs. *Antagonism*: The addition of a second drug decreases the effectiveness of the first. *Indifferent*: No interaction between the drugs. The calculation is aided by an isobologram graph. This facilitates visual evaluation of the interaction but requires a separate statistical analysis. The isobolographic analysis for the MIC is more sensitive because the analysis evaluates the dose effects and is the prelude to studies in *in vivo* pharmacodynamics [86].

In coinfections, patients are exposed to simultaneous antifungal and antibacterial therapeutic treatment. Quinolones and antifungals are commonly used in bacteria and fungi or bacteria and yeast coinfections. Nakajima *et. al.*, reported the synergistic effect of DU-9859a fluoroquinolone enhanced the *in vitro* antifungal activity of amphothericin B and fluconazole against *Candida* spp. growth and decreased the load in mice infected with yeast. The last result was also observed in mice infected with *Aspergillus fumigatus* [87]. Similar results were obtained with ciprofloxacin, amphotericin B, levofloxacin, voriconazole, or caspofungin combinations, which has a synergistic effect against *Candida albicans* and *Aspergillus fumigatus* [88]. In another report, ofloxacin had a synergic effect on fluconazole versus a fluconazole-resistant *Candida albicans* strain [89].

Analysis of drug interactions with simultaneous application is still developing. Modified methods have been proposed related to more accurate isobolographic analysis, and *in vitro* models approach physiological conditions. Animal models have also been used. This area will revolutionize therapeutic interventions.

19. Biofilms

An appreciation for the fact that in nature bacteria adhere to many abiotic or biotic surfaces, embedded in an extracellular matrix, and form communities known as "biofilms" has emerged over the past few decades [90]. Biofilm formation conferred on individual bacteria the ability to collaborate and to adapt to a range of harsh environmental conditions and, perhaps most of all, to evade predation by phagocytic microbes. The formation of a biofilm provides a microbe with a small measure of control over the local environment, including fluctuations in temperature, pH, ultraviolet light, starvation, and exposure to toxic agents [91, 92].

Advances in medical biofilm research have led to the understanding that biofilms represent the prevalent form of bacterial life during tissue colonization and may occur in more than 80 % of microbial infections in the body [93].

Members of a biofilm community, which can be of the same or multiple species, show varying stages of differentiation and exchange information, metabolites, and genes with each other. As a result, members of the biofilm community are in a diversity of physiologies influenced by the unequal sharing of nutrients and metabolic by-products, which results in subpopulations with increased tolerance to antimicrobials and environmental stresses, the host immune system, and predatory microorganisms [19, 94, 95, 96, 97, 98].

Canonically, biofilm development has been grouped into five stages that are reflective of conditions in many, but not all, biofilms: (1) reversible aggregation of planktonic cells on a surface, (2) irreversible adhesion, (3) formation of microcolonies, (4) biofilm maturation, and (5) detachment and dispersion of cells [99]. The events that are of special significance for ocular infections and the treatment of biofilm infections will be discussed in greater detail, while the reader is referred to several excellent reviews for details on other biofilm-related subjects [19, 100,101].

The biofilms involve the production of an extracellular matrix (ECM) that embedded the cells and, in some cases, binds the cells together and that can be composed of polysaccharides, lipopolysaccharides, proteins, or extracellular DNA [10]. This process may be active or passive, in that cells on the surface of an adherent colony that are lysed by the ejection of neutrophil antimicrobial factors may encase and protect siblings below in a matrix consisting simply of cell lysate. Whatever the nature of the matrix, its chemical and physical properties contribute to the differentiation of cells within the encased population, a process that can protect the bacteria from the action of antimicrobial agents, host immune responses, bacteriophages, and phagocytic amoeba [19].

http://dx.doi.org/10.5772/64702

As the microcolony grows through cell division or the recruitment of more planktonic cells, the biofilm grows and takes on a three-dimensional structure that often includes open water channels [19, 103].

The three-dimensional organization of the biofilm causes gradients of oxygen, pH, and nutrients, resulting in the development of different microniches [104, 105, 106]. The cell's individual physiological adaptations to these microniches result in physiological heterogeneity [98]. Cells near the surface of the biofilm will be exposed to more nutrients and oxygen and are therefore more metabolically active, while cells in the deep regions will be less active or even dormant. This heterogeneity results in a range of responses to antimicrobial agents, with metabolically active cells at the surface being rapidly killed, while more internal, dormant cells are comparatively unaffected [106]. This, together with potential effects on the diffusion of antimicrobial molecules within the biofilm, causes some cells in a biofilm to be recalcitrant to antimicrobial treatment, with antibiotic susceptibilities reduced by 10- to 1,000-fold compared to their planktonic counterparts [106].

The high local concentration of cells in a biofilm creates an ideal environment for information exchange through cell-to-cell communication and lateral gene transfer. Cell signaling mediated by secreted, accumulating messenger molecules, known as quorum sensing, allows bacteria to sense and respond to their environment and couple cell density and other environmental cues with gene expression in ways that allow adaptive phenotypic responses. Quorum sensing has been shown to be involved in the control of biofilm formation and the production of virulence and colonization factors in a variety of organisms of medical importance [106]. Cell-to-cell signaling is also involved in biofilm dispersion, which is of general and medical interest [107].

20. Practical strategies for coinfection diagnosis

The two leading causes of vision impairment worldwide are uncorrected refractive errors and cataract. Measures for managing those eye abnormalities frequently include the use of contact lenses and the placement of intraocular lenses and have enhanced the quality of life of millions of patients. Although the use of such devices is the great importance for correction of a variety of visual aberrations, these devices also provide a new surface on which many microbial pathogens can form biofilms (Table 2). As a result, device-related ocular infections are an important limitation of the success of such procedures. Moreover, many infections progress to secondary permanent sequelae that may lead to poor visual outcomes and occasionally loss of sight, such as acute bacterial endophthalmitis or corneal ulceration.

In all infection diseases, not only ocular infection, it is important to make sure of the microbiological diagnosis, especially when the coinfections are a large percentage of the total infections. The results will provide a report on the distribution and trends in microbiological and antibiotic sensitivity patterns that will affect the patient's treatment and prognosis. We have developed simple and practical strategies in each phase for ocular infection diagnosis, including the coinfections summarized in Figure 1.

Disease	Main causative agents of infection and/or found in the biofilms	Biofilm localization
Endophthalmitis	Coagulase-negative staphylococci and *Propionibacterium acnes*	Intraocular lens posterior capsule
Keratitis	*Staphylococcus aureus* and other staphylococcal species, *Pseudomonas aeruginosa* and *Serratia* spp. Fungi and *Acanthamoeba* spp. less frequently	Contact lens
	Viridans group Streptococci. Gram-negative bacilli and yeasts less frequently	Corneal stroma (crystalline keratopathy)
Scleral buckle infection	Gram-positive cocci and nontuberculous *Mycobacterium* spp.	Scleral buckles
Lacrimal system infections	*Staphylococcus* spp., *P. aeruginosa,* and *M. chelonae*	Lacrimal intubation devices
	Staphylococcus spp.	Punctual plugs
Periorbital infections	*Staphylococcus* spp. and mixed species biofilms	Sockets and orbital plates

Table 2. Biofilm-associated infections of the eye

A successful microbiological study consists in a correct identification, but, it begins since the pre-analytic phase, where the ophthalmologist plays an important role, so that, in our laboratory, we have improved an initial lesson to emphasize two principal things. The first thing is awareness of the importance to take the ocular sample before the intensive topical antibiotic treatment. It allows us to have greater chance of bacterial growth, although it has been described that scraping may accelerate disease resolution by enhancing antibiotic penetration and the therapeutic debridement of the necrotic tissue [108]. The second thing is that during the lesson we teach to the ophthalmologist the properly way to select, collect, and transport the sample to optimize the analysis and interpretation. For the collection, we prepared kits with all the necessary to take the sample for a molecular and microbiological diagnosis; the kit contains chocolate agar (ChA), Columbia agar (CA), and Brain-Heart Infusion (BHI); these are enrichment mediums for the exigent bacteria growth, like *Streptococcus* spp. and *Kocuria* spp.; the kit also contains Sabouraud dextrose agar (SDA), for fungi growth; different types of applicators (cotton, alginate, and rayon), a glass slide for the frotis, and finally a transport media for the molecular diagnosis are also included. On the other hand, we have accord with the ophthalmologist the conditions for the sample collection and storage that are summarized in Table 3, and especially, we have established the sequence for seeded the sample because of the small amount of material and small numbers of organisms obtainable from the eye: one swab for ChA, CA, and BHI, another swab for SDA, and the frotis for Gram, Wright, and Calcofluor stain. In conclusion, the pre-analytic phase is a continuous team work between the ophthalmologist and the laboratory staff.

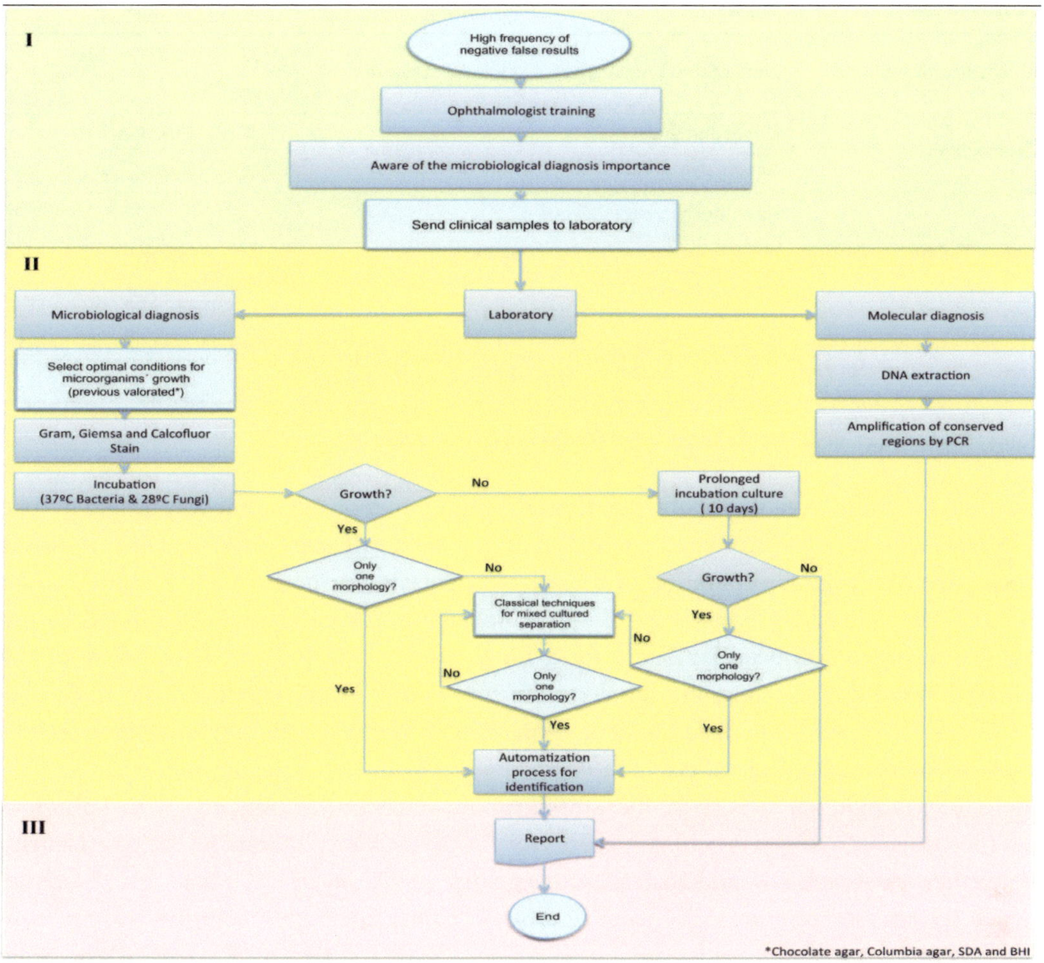

Figure 1. Practical strategies for coinfection diagnosis during the three analytic phases. (I) The pre-analytic phase, when the ophthalmologist is training for selecting, collecting, and transporting the sample, plays an important role. (II) The analytic phase with microbiological and molecular techniques. In the microbiological diagnosis, the laboratory staff's experience is important to discern a pure from a mixed culture; molecular techniques are used to determine non-cultivable microorganisms. (III) The post-analytic phase, the final result in which the partnership between the ophthalmologist and the laboratory staff is reflected in the best outcomes for patients.

In the analytic phase, the sample could be processed by microbiology or by molecular techniques. About the microbiological diagnosis, the agar plates are checked every day, looking for bacterial or fungal growth. We have implemented a prolonged microorganism cultured of up to 15 days, because most of the hospital population includes multi-treatment patients, so that the microorganisms begin to grow until a week of incubation. Most of the times, the microorganisms involved in a coinfection are closely interacting, being impossible the identification in the automatized system (Vitek 2C, bioMérieux, France). The use of simple and classical microbiological techniques has allowed us to separate these interactions, for

Ocular infection	Sample	Equipment	Storage conditions
Keratitis/corneal ulcer	Limit of the corneal ulcer	Alginate applicator	37 °C→ChA, CA, BHI 28 °C→SDA
Conjunctivitis	Upper and lower eyelid conjunctiva	Cotton applicator	37 °C→ChA, CA, BHI 28 °C→SDA
Endophthalmitis and uveitis	Anterior chamber (aqueous humor)	Sterile syringes	4 °C→ syringes
	Vitreous humor		

Chocolate agar (ChA), Columbia agar (CA), Brain-Heart Infusion (BHI), Sabouraud dextrose agar (SDA), 37 °C for bacteria growth, 28 °C for fungi growth, and 4 °C for sample conservation

Table 3. Conditions for the sample collection and storage from ocular infections

example, the sonication (physical separation technique based on ultrasonic waves) and the use of selective media as MacConkey agar (MCk) and mannitol-salt agar (MSA) seeded by a perfect open streak for a good separation of the microorganisms, for positive and negative Gram bacteria, respectively. Talking about the fungi infections, the good sample collected by the ophthalmologists has been sufficient for a fungi growth and a direct observation of the macromorphology and micromorphology for the identification. However, the molecular techniques have revolutionized the ocular infection and coinfection diagnosis; these techniques are more sensitive, specific, and rapid and impact in the best outcome for the patient. The molecular techniques consist in the amplification of conserved regions of the different microorganisms involved in ocular infection, for example, Gram (+)/Gram (−) bacteria; Generic Fungi; herpes viruses I, II, and zoster; Cytomegalovirus; *Chlamydia* sp.; adenovirus; *Mycobacterium tuberculosis* complex (MTC) and no *Mycobacterium tuberculosis* complex (NTC); *Toxoplasma gondii*; and *Acanthamoeba* spp. by polymerase chain reaction (PCR). The PCR helps us for the identification of coinfection caused not only bacteria-bacteria or bacteria-fungi but also coinfection caused by viruses and parasites with bacteria or fungi.

Finally, the post-analytic phase consists of the interpretation of the results. Most laboratories do not report *Staphylococcus epidermidis* and *Staphylococcus aureus*, because they are part of the ocular surface microbiota; however, the laboratory staff of ocular microbiology knows that these microorganisms can be involved directly in the ocular infection, and these two microorganisms have been reported as the microorganisms most frequently isolated in infectious keratitis [109, 110]. It is important to consider the risk factor associated before deciding whether the microorganisms isolated are responsible for the infection or are a contamination.

In conclusion, the diagnosis of infectious disease is best achieved by applying in-depth knowledge of medical and laboratory science by integrating a strategic view of host-parasite interactions. Clearly, the best outcomes for patients are the result of strong partnerships between the clinician and the laboratory specialist [111].

21. Conclusion

The relationship between microorganisms has a long evolutionary history. The ability of microorganisms to interact conferred the possibility to collaborate and to adapt within a wider spectrum of environmental conditions. These circumstances have a direct impact on the clinical presentation as well as the dynamics of infection in the population.

Delay in diagnosis affects the sensitivity to specific treatments and the evolution of infection. The rate of recovery could be slow and morbid, leaving serious sequelae with the risk of loss of vision. Advances in methods for detecting infectious organisms and molecular microbiology have facilitated the recognition of the interactions among pathogens found in coinfections in the human eye. The acute period of coinfection is determinant to identify the coinfecting microorganisms. Awareness in the medical field and particularly in ophthalmology of lesions that do not cover the conditions of a pathognomonic clinical picture should be resolved with molecular biology techniques together with classical techniques of microorganism recognition, until final identification, if possible.

In this chapter, we proposed a strategy for reducing the uncertainty of the presence of two or more microorganisms affecting the eye. This has been implemented in our laboratory and has increased the possibility of isolation and identification.

In addition, the biofilm of each combination of pathogens must be studied molecularly to understand its particular adhesion and aggregation, possible mutations, and strategies for evasion or elimination of antimicrobial. Together with pharmacodynamics, *in vivo* studies will facilitate the application of different antimicrobial dosages to successfully remove coinfecting microorganisms.

Author details

Carlos Alberto Pantoja-Meléndez[1,2*], Victor M. Bautista-de Lucio[1], Mariana Ortiz-Casas[1], Jonathan Quevedo-Martínez[1] and Herlinda Mejía-López[1]

*Address all correspondence to: linda.mejia@institutodeoftalmologia.org

1 Institute of Opthalmology Conde de Valenciana, Mexico

2 National Autonomous University of Mexico, School of Medicine, Public Health Department, Mexico

References

[1] Whitcher J, Srinivasan M. "Corneal blindness: a global perspective". Bull World Health Organ. 2001; 79: p. 214-221.

[2] Birger R, Kouyos R, Cohen T, Griffiths S, Huijben S, Mina M, *et. al*. The potential impact of coinfection on antimicrobial chemotherapy and drug resistance. Trends Microbiol. 2015; 15: p. 106-107.

[3] Frey-Klett P, Burlinson P, Deveau A, Barret M, Tarkka M, Sarniguet A. Bacterial-Fungal Interactions: Hyphens between Agricultural, Clinical, Environmental, and Food Microbiologists. Microbiol Mol Biol Rev. 2011 Dec; 75 (4): 583–609

[4] Russler S, Tapper M, Knox K, Liepins A, Carrigan D. Pneumonitis associated with coinfection by human herpesvirus 6 and Legionella in an immunocompetent adult. Am J Pathol. 1991; 138: p. 1405-1411.

[5] Day T, Graham A, A R. Evolution of parasite virulence when host responses cause disease. Proc Biol Sci. 2007; 274: p. 2685-2692.

[6] Jindal A, Moreker M, Pathengay A, Khera M, Jalali A, Majji A, *et. al*. Polymicrobial endophthalmitis: prevalence, causative organisms, and visual outcomes. J Ophtalmic Inflamm Infect. 2013; 3: p. 6.

[7] Iwalokun B, Oluwadum A, Akisinde K, Niemogha M, Nwaokorie F. Bacteriologic and plasmid analysis of etiologic agents of conjunctivitis in Lagos, Nigeria. J Ophthalmic Inflamm Infect. 2011; 3: p. 95-103.

[8] Huang Y, Yang B, Li W. Defining the normal core microbiome of conjunctival microbial communities. Clin Microbiol Infect. 2016; 16: p. 30065-30069.

[9] Lim N, Lim D, Ray M. Polymicrobial versus monomicrobial keratitis: a retrospective comparative study. Eye Contact Lens. 2013; 39: p. 348-354.

[10] Gopinathan U, Sharma S, Garg P, Rao G. Review of epidemiological features, microbiological diagnosis and treatment outcome of microbial keratitis: experience of over a decade. Indian J Opthalmol. 2009; 57: p. 273-279.

[11] Basak S, Mohanta A, Bhowmick A. Epidemiological and microbiological diagnosis of suppurative keratitis in Gangetic West Bengal, eastern India. Indian J Ophthalmol. 2005; 53: p. 17-22.

[12] Bharathi M, Ramakrishnan R, Vasu R, Meenakshi PR. Aetiological diagnosis of microbial keratitis in South India - A study of 1618 cases. Indian J Med Microbiol. 2002; 20: p. 19-24.

[13] Jones D. Polymicrobial keratitis. Tr Am Ophth Soc. 1981; 79: p. 153-157.

[14] Brand A, Barnes J, K M, Odds F, Gow N. Cell wall glycans and soluble factors determine the interactions between the hyphae of Candida albicans and Pseudomonas aeruginosa. FEMS Microbiol Lett. 2008; 287: p. 48-55.

[15] Seidler M, Salvenmoser S, Muller F. Aspergillus fumigatus forms biofilms with reduced antifungal drug susceptibility on bronchial epithelial cells. Antimicrob Agents Chemother. 2008; 52: p. 4130-4136.

[16] Loussert C, Schmitt C, Prevost M. In vivo biofilm composition of Aspergillus fumigatus. Cell MIcrobiol. 2010; 12: p. 405-410.

[17] Mah T, O'Toole G. Mechanisms of biofilm resistance to antimicrobial agents. Trens Microbiol. 2001; 9: p. 34-39.

[18] Steward P, Costerton J. Antibiotic resistance of bacteria in biofilms. Lancet. 2001; 14: p. 135-138.

[19] Kıvanç SA, Kıvanç M, Bayramlar H. Microbiology of corneal wounds after cataract surgery: biofilm formation and antibiotic resistance patterns. J Wound Care. 2016; 25: 12: p. 14-19.

[20] Fröhlich S, Miño de Kaspar H, Grasbon T, Möhring C, Klauss V, Kampik A. Bacterial keratitis. Microbiological analysis as a principle for therapeutic recommendations. Pphthalmologe. 1999; 7: p. 459-464.

[21] Yeh D, Stinnett S, Afshari N. Analysis of bacterial cultures in infectious keratitis, 1997 to 2004. Am J Opthalmol. 2006; 6: p. 1066-1068.

[22] Kim J, H S, Song J. Infectious keratitis caused by Stenotrophomonas maltophilia and yeast simultaneously. Cornea. 2006; 10: p. 1234-1236.

[23] Qiu W, Yao Y. Mycotic keratitis caused by concurrent infections of Exserohilum mcginnisii and Candida parapsilosis. BMC Ophthalmol. 2013; 13: p. 37-40.

[24] Katragkou A, Z P, Perlin D, Kontoyiannis D, Walsh T, Roilides E. Exserohilum infection Review of 48 cases before the 2012 United States outbreak. The pediatric Infectious Disease Journal. 2005; 24: p. 939-941.

[25] Yokoi N, Okada K, Sugita J, Kinoshita S. Acute conjunctivitis associated with biofilm formation on a punctal plug. Jpn J Opthalmol. 2000; 44: p. 559-560.

[26] Taff HMK, Edward J, Andes D. Mechanisms of Candida biofilm drug resistance. Future Microbiol. 2013; 8: p. 1325-1337.

[27] Hayashi Y, Eguchi H, Toibana T, Mitamura Y, Yaguchi T. Polymicrobial sclerokeratitis caused by Scedosporium apiospermum and Aspergillus cibarius. Cornea. 2014; 33: p. 875-877.

[28] Schuster F, Visvesvara G. Free-living amoebae as opportunistic and non-opportunistic pathogens of human and animals. Int J Parasitol. 2004; 34: p. 1001-1027.

[29] Galarza C, Gutiérrez E, Uribe M, Ramos W, Ortega A, Ávila J, *et. al*. Amebas de vida libre en lesiones cutaneas. Reporte de 4 casos. Dermatol Perú. 2006; 16: p. 36-40.

[30] Scheid P. Relevance of free-living amoebae as hosts for phylogenetically diverse microorganisms. parasitol Res. 2014; 113: p. 2407-2414.

[31] Barker J, Lambert P, Brown M. Influence of intra-amoebic and other growth conditions on the surface properties of Legionella pneumophila. Infec Immun. 1993; 61: p. 3503-3510.

[32] Lim N, Goh D, Bunce C, Xing W, Fraenkel G, Poole T, *et. al.* Comparison of polyhexamethylene biguanide and chlorhexidine as monotherapy agents in the treatment of Acanthamoeba keratitis. Am J Ophthalmol. 2008; 145: p. 130-135.

[33] Scheid P. Mechanism of intrusion of a microspordian-like organism into the nucleus of host amoebae (Vannella sp.) isolated from a keratitis patient. Parasitol Res. 2007; 101: p. 1097-1102.

[34] Scheid P, Hauroder B, Michel R. Investigations of an extraordinary endocytobiont in Acanthamoeba sp., development and replication. Parasitol Res. 2010; 106: p. 1371-1377.

[35] Qureshi M, Perez A, Madayag R, Bottone E. Inhibition of Acanthamoeba species by Pseudomonas aeruginosa: rationale for their selective exclusion in corneal ulcers and contact lens care systems. J Clin Microbiol. 1993; 31: p. 1908-1910.

[36] Bottone E, R M, Qureshi M. Acanthamoeba keratitis: synergy between amebic and bacterial cocontaminants in contact lens care systems as a prelude to infection. J Clin Microbiol. 1992; 30: p. 2447-2450.

[37] Lorenzo-Morales J, Khan N, Walochnik J. An update on Acanthamoeba keratitis: diagnosis, pathogenesis and treatment. Parasite. 2015; 22: p. 10.

[38] Sharma R, Jhanji V, Satpathy G, Sharma N, Khokhar S, Agarwal T. Coinfection with Acanthamoeba and Pseudomonas in contact lens-associated keratitis. Optom Vis Sci. 2013; 90: p. 53-55.

[39] Michel R, Hauroder B. Isolation of an Acanthamoeba strain with intracellular Burkholderia pickettii infection. Zentralbl Bakteriol. 1997; 285: p. 541-547.

[40] Mauger T, Craig E. Combined acanthamoeba and Stenotrophomonas maltophilia keratitis treated with a conjunctival flap followed by penetrating keratoplasty. Cornea. 2006; 25: p. 631-633.

[41] Hong J, Ji J, Xu J, Cao W, Liu Z, Sun X. An unusual case of Acanthamoeba Polyphaga and Pseudomonas Aeruginosa keratitis. Diagn Pathol. 2014; 9: p. 105.

[42] Lone R, Syed K, Abdul R, Sheikh S, Shah F. Unusual case of methicillin resistant staphylococcus aureus and Acanthamoeba keratitis in a non-contact lens wearer from Kashmir, India. BMJ Case Re. 2009; p. 8.

[43] Dini L, Cockinos C, Frean J, Niszl I, Markus M. Unusual case of acanthamoeba polyphaga and Pseudomonas aeruginosa keratitis in a contact lens wearer from Gauteng, South Africa. L Clin Microbiol. 2000; 38: p. 826-829.

[44] Tu E, Joslin C, Nijm L, Feder R, Jain S, Shoff M. Polymicrobial keratitis: Acanthamoeba and infectious crystalline keratopathy. Am J Ophthalmol. 2009; 148: p. 13.

[45] Gupta S, Shrivastava R, tandom R, Gogia V, Agarwal P, Satpathy G. Role of voriconazole in combined acanthamoeba and fungal corneal ulcer. Cont Lnes Anterior Eye. 2011; 34: p. 287-289.

[46] Rumelt S, Cohen I, Lefler E, Rehany U. Corneal co-infection with Scedosporium apiospermum and Acanthamoeba after sewage-contaminated ocular injury. Cornea. 2001; 20: p. 112-116.

[47] Tien S, Sheu M. Treatment of Acanthamoeba keratitis combined with fungal infection with polyhexamethylene biguanide. Kaohsiung J Med Sci. 1999; 15: p. 665-673.

[48] Froumis N, Mondino B, Glaswow B. Acanthamoeba keratitis associated with fungal keratitis. Eye Contact Lens. 2008; 34: p. 185-187.

[49] Slade D, Johnson J, Tabin G. Acanthamoeba and fungal keratitis in a woman with a history of Intacs corneal implants. Eye Contact Lens. 2008; 34: p. 185-187.

[50] Dong Q, Brulc J, Iovieno A, Bates B GA, Miller D, Revanna K, *et. al*. Diversity of bacteria at healthy human conjunctiva. Invest Ophthalmol Vis Sci. 2011; 52: p. 5408-5413.

[51] Dalfré J, Rodrigues J, Donato B, Giancoli A, De Carvalho J, De Andrade D, *et. al*. Fungic microbiota of normal conjunctiva, sugar-cane and anemophilous fungi of the region of Monte Belo- Minas Gerais. Arq Bras Oftalmol. 2007; 70: p. 445-449.

[52] Moreno N, Moreno R, Sousa L. Aerobic bacterial microbiota of the conjunctiva in diabetic patients with normal and altered glycated hemoglobin levels in two regions in Brazil. Arq Bras Oftalmol. 2014; 77: p. 351-354.

[53] Schabereiter-Gurtner C, Maca S, Rölleke S, Nigl K, Lukas J, Hirschl A, *et. al*. 16S rDNA-based identification of bacteria from conjunctival swabs by PCR and DGGE fingerprinting. Invest Ophthalmol Vis Sci. 2001; 42: p. 1164-1171.

[54] Tappe D, Mueller A, WeiBbrich B, Schubert J, Schargus M, Stich A. Severe conjunctivitis due to multidrug-resistant Neisseria gonorrhoeae and adenovirus 53 coinfection in a traveler returning from Thailand. J Travel Med. 2013; 20: p. 403-406.

[55] Mellman-Rubin T, Kowaski R, Uhrin M, Gordon Y. Incidence of adenoviral and chlamydial coinfection in acute follicular conjunctivitis. 1995; 119: p. 652-654.

[56] Galvis V, Tello A, Guerra A, Acuña M, Villarreal D. Antibiotic susceptibility patterns of bacteria isolated from keratitis and intraocular infections at Fundación Oftalmológica de Santander (FOSCAL. Florida Blanca Colombia Biomedica. 2014; 34: p. 23-33.

[57] Gupta A, Gupta V, Dogra M, Panday S, Ray P. Chkraborty A. Spectrum and clinical profile of post cataract surgery endophthalmitis in north India. Indian J Ophthalmol. 2003;51: p.139-145.

[58] Pijl B, Theelen T, Tilanus M, Rentenaar R, Crama N. Acute endophthalmitis after cataract surgery: 250 consecutive cases treated at a tertiary referral center in the Netherlands. Am J Ophthalmol. 2010; 149: p. 482-487.

[59] Gharamah AA, Moharram AM, Ismail MA, Al-Hussaini AK. Bacterial and fungal endophthalmitis in upper Egypt: related species and risk factors. Asian Pac J Trop Biomed. 2012; 2: p. 655-659.

[60] Kunimoto D, Das T, Sharma S, Jalali S, Majji A, Gopinathan U, *et. al.* Microbiologic spectrum and susceptibility of isolates: part II. Posttraumatic endophthalmitis. Endophthalmitis Research Group. Am J Ophthalmol. 1999; 128: p. 242-244.

[61] Long C, Liu B, Xu C, Jing Y, Yuan Z, Lin X. Causative organisms of post-traumatic endophthalmitis: a 20-year retrospective study. BMC Ophthlmol. 2014; 25: p. 34.

[62] Duan F, Wu K, Liao J, Zheng Y, Yuan Z, Tan J, Lin X. Causative Microorganisms of Infectious Endophthalmitis: A 5-Year Retrospective Study. J Ophthalmol. 2016; 2016: 1-7.

[63] Streilen J. Ocular immune privilege: the eye takes a dim but practical view of immunity and inflammation. J Leukoc Biol. 2003; 74: p. 179-185.

[64] Matricardi P, Rosmini F, Riondino S, Fortini M, Ferrigno L, Rapicetta M, *et. al.*Exposure to foodborne and orofecal microbes versus airborne viruses in relation to atopy and allergic asthma: epidemiological study. BMJ. 2000; 320: p. 412-417.

[65] Kurata A. Hygiene hypothesis: why south/north geographical differences in prevalence of asthma and sarcoidosis? Med Hypotheses. 2012; 79: p. 363-364.

[66] von Hertzen LC. Puzzling associations between childhood infections and the later occurrence of asthma and atopy. Ann Med. 2000; 32: p. 397-400.

[67] Kerr N, Stern G. Bacterial keratitis associated with vernal keratoconjunctivitis. Cornea. 1992; 11: p. 355-359.

[68] Rolinski J, Hus I. Immunological aspects of acute and recurrent herpes simplex keratitis. J Immunol Res. 2014; p. 51.

[69] Stric L, Wald A, Celum C. Management of herpes simplex virus type 2 infection in HIV type 1-infected persons. Clin Infec Dis. 2006; 43: p. 347-356.

[70] Faber D, Wiley C, Lynn G, Gross J, Freeman W. Role of HIV and CMV in the pathogenesis of retinitis and retinal vasculopathy in AIDS patients. Invest Ophthalmol Vis Sci. 1992; 33: p. 2345-2353.

[71] Radu L, Serban R, Cornăcel C, Cioboata M, Anghel A. Cytomegalovirus retinitis in HIV/AIDS patients. J Med Life. 2014; 15: p. 237-240.

[72] Freigassner P, Ardjomand N, Radner H, El-Shabrawi Y. Coinfection of the retina by Epstein-Barr virus and cytomegalovirus in an AIDS patient. Am J Opthalmol. 2002; 134: p. 275-257.

[73] Skolnik P, Pomerantz R, De la Monte S, Lee S, Hsiung G, Foos R, *et. al.* Dual infection of retina with human immunodeficiency virus type 1 and cytomegalovirus. Am J Ophthalmol. 1989; 107: p. 361-372.

[74] Rummelt V, Rummelt C, Jahn G, Wenkel H, Sinzger C, Mayer U, *et. al.* Triple retinal infection with human immunodeficiency virus type 1, cytomegalovirus, and herpes simplex virus type 1. Light and electron microscopy, immunohistochemistry, and in situ hybridization. Ophthalmology. 1994; 101: p. 270-279.

[75] Kim J, Singer E, Bonelli L, Klausner J. A case of primary HIV type 1 and cytomegalovirus coinfection presenting with widespread clinical disease. J Int Assoc Provid AIDS Care. 2014; 13: p. 196-199.

[76] Matoba A. Polymicrobial keratitis secondary to Burkholderia ambifaria, enterococcus, and staphylococcus aureus in a patient with herpetic stromal keratitis. Am J Ophthalmol. 2003; 136: p. 748-749.

[77] Tandon R, Vajpayee R, Gupta V, Vajpayee M, Satpathy G, Dada T. Polymicrobial keratitis in an HIV-positive patient. Indian J Ophthalmol. 2003; 51: p. 87-88.

[78] Wayne P. Reference Method for Broth dilution antifungal susceptibility testing of filamentous fungi. 2nd ed. USA; 2008.

[79] Abdelillah A, Houcine B, Halima D, Meriem C, Imane Z, Eddine S, *et. al.* Evaluation of antifungal activity of free fatty acids methyl esters fraction isolated from Algerian Linum usitatissimum L. seeds against toxigenic Aspergillus. Asian Pac J Trop Biomed. 2013; 3: p. 443-448.

[80] Ponce D, Bautista-de-Lucio V, Santacrúz-Valdés C, Climent-Flores A, Rodríguez-Tovar A, Robles-Contreras A, *et. al.* Effect of simultaneous treatment of quinolones and antifungal drugs on fungal-bacterial coculture. In ARVO 2012.

[81] Pradhan L, Sharma S, Nalamada S, Sahu S, DS, Garg P. Natamycin in the treatment of keratomycosis: correlation of treatment outcome and in vitro susceptibility of fungal isolates. Indian J Ophthalmol. 2011; 59: p. 512-514.

[82] Pate J, Jones D, Wilhelmus K. Prevalence and spectrum of bacterial co-infection during fungal keratitis. Br J Opthalmol. 2006; 90: p. 289-292.

[83] Mosquera J, Denning D. Azole cross-resistance in Aspergillus fumigatus. Antimicrob Agents Chemother. 2002; 46: p. 556-557.

[84] Hanet M, Jamart J, Chaves A. Fluoroquinolones or fortified antibiotics for treating bacterial keratitis: systematic review and meta-analysis of comparative studies. Can J Ophthalmol. 2012; 47: p. 493-499.

[85] Jin K, Jeon H, Hyon J, Wee W, Suh W, Shin Y, *et. al*. A case of fungal keratitis and onychomycosis simultaneously infected by Trichophyton species. BMC. 2014; 11: p. 37 90.

[86] Tallarida R. Drug synergism: its detection and applications. J Pharmacol Exp Ther. 2001; 298: p. 865-872.

[87] Nakajima R, Kitamura A, Someya K, Tanaka M, Sato K. In vitro and in vivo antifungal activities of DU-6859a, a fluoroquinolone, in combination with amphotericin B and fluconazole against pathogenic fungi. Antimicrob Agents Chemother. 1995; 39: p. 1517-1521.

[88] Stergiopoulou T, Meletiadis J, Sein T, Papaioannidou P, Tsiouris I, Roilides E, *et. al*. Comparative pharmacodynamic interaction analysis between ciprofloxacin, moxifloxacin and levofloxacin and antifungal agents against Candida albicans and Aspergillus fumigatus. J Antimicrob Chemother. 2009; 63: p. 343-348.

[89] Sasaki E, Maesaki S, Miyazaki Y, Yanagihara K, Tomono K, Tashiro T, *et. al*. Synergistic effect of ofloxacin and fluconazole against azole-resistant Candida albicans. J Infec Chemother. 2000; 6: p. 151-154.

[90] Costerton J, Geesey G, Cheng K. How bacteria stick. Sci Am. 1978; 238: p. 86-95.

[91] Hall-Stoodley L, Costerton J, Stoodley P. Bacterial biofilms: From the natural environment to infectious diseases. Nat Rev Microbiol. 2004; 2: p. 95-108.

[92] Harrison J, Ceri H, Turner R. Multimetal resistance and tolerance in microbial biofilms. Nat Rev Microbiol. 2007; 5: p. 928-938.

[93] Health. NIo. Research on microbial biofilms (PA-03-047). [Online] . 2002; [cited 2015 January 10.] Available from: HYPERLINK "http://grants.nih.gov/grants/guide/pafiles/PA-03-047.html"http://grants.nih.gov/grants/guide/pa-files/PA-03-047.html.

[94] Donlan R, Costerton J. Biofilms: Survival mechanisms of clinically relevant microorganisms. Clin Microbiol Rev. 2002; 15: p. 167-193.

[95] Annous B, Fratamico P, Smith J. Scientific status summary. J Food Sci. 2009; 74: p. R24-37.

[96] Hooshangi S, Bentley W. From unicellular properties to multicellular behavior: Bacteria quorum sensing circuitry and applications. Curr Opin Biotechnol. 2008; 19: p. 550-555.

[97] Stewart P, Franklin M. Physiological heterogeneity in biofilms. Nat Rev Microbiol. 2008; 6: p. 199-210.

[98] Watnick P, Kolter R. Biofilm, city of microbes. J Bacteriol. 2000; 182: p. 2675-2679.

[99] Fux CA, Costerton JW, Stewart PS, Stoodley P. Survival strategies of infectious biofilms. Trends Microbiol. 2005; 13: p. 34-40.

[100] Costerton J, Stewart P, biofilms B. Battling biofilms. Sci Am. 2001; 285: p. 74-81.

[101] Behlau I, Gilmore M. Microbial biofilms in ophthalmology and infectious disease. Arch Ophthalmol. 2008; 126: p. 1572-1581.

[102] H, Wingender J. The biofilm matrix. Nat Rev Microbiol. 2010; 8: p. 623-633.

[103] Sauer K, Camper A, Ehrlich G, Costerton J, Davies D. Pseudomonas aeruginosa displays multiple phenotypes during development as a biofilm. J Bacteriol. 2002; 184: p. 1140-1154.

[104] Hall-Stoodley L, Stoodley P. Evolving concepts in biofilm infections. Cell Microbiol. 2009; 11: p. 1034-1043.

[105] Davies D. Understanding biofilm resistance to antibacterial agents. Nat Rev Drug Discov. 2003; 2: p. 114-122.

[106] Spoering A, Gilmore M. Quorum sensing and DNA release in bacterial biofilms. Curr Opin Microbiol. 2006; 9: p. 133-137.

[107] Kaplan J. Biofilm dispersal: Mechanisms, clinical implications, and potential therapeutic uses. J Dent Res. 2010; 89: p. 205-218.

[108] Allan B, Garth J. Strategies for the management of microbial keratitis. Br J Ophthalmol. 1995; 79: p. 777-786.

[109] Hernandez-Camarena JC, Graue-Hernandez EO, Ortiz-Casas M, Ramirez-Miranda A, Navas A, Pedro-Aguilar L, *et al.* Trends in Microbiological and Antibiotic Sensitivity Patterns in Infectious Keratitis: 10-Year Experience in Mexico City. Cornea. 2015; 34: p. 778-785.

[110] Lichtinger A, Yeung S, Kim P. Shifting trends in bacterial keratitis in Toronto: an 11-18 year review. Ophthalmology. 2012; 119: p. 1785-1790.

[111] Baron E, Miller M, Weinstein M. A Guide to Utilization of the Microbiology Laboratory for Diagnosis of Infectious Diseases: 2013 Recommendations by the Infectious Diseases Society of America (IDSA) and the American Society for Microbiology; 2013.

Section 3

Miscellaneous Issues

Chapter 6

The Risk of Infection in Dry Eye Syndrome Accompanying Primary Sjögren's Syndrome

Maria Maślińska and Brygida Kwiatkowska

Additional information is available at the end of the chapter

http://dx.doi.org/10.5772/64243

Abstract

Primary Sjögren's syndrome (pSS) is an autoimmune disease, which dominates the symptoms resulting from inflammatory infiltrates in exocrine glands. Frequently, patients complain of a feeling of sand under the eyelids, eye irritation, and red eye caused by a decrease in tear secretion. The ophthalmic examination beyond lowering the secretion of tears in Schirmer's test evaluation in cases with a significant intensification of dry eye disease (DED) can be visualized by measuring ocular staining score (OSS) using lissamine green and fluorescein staining. OSS can demonstrate the degree of damage to the corneal surface. It is known that keratoconjunctivitis sicca (KCS) in pSS is not only limited to the complaints of unpleasant feeling of sand under the eyelids but also can lead to serious corneal damage and decreased vision even to blindness. And between the others, complications of KCS in pSS must be replaced with an increased susceptibility to infection. We should also pay attention to possible co-infection with Epstein-Barr virus (EBV) virus and bacterial co-infections, e.g., *Chlamydia pneumoniae, Staphylococcus aureus,* or latent conjunctival infections *Chlamydia trachomatis, Mycoplasma hominis,* and *Ureaplasma urealyticum* in group of patients with DED, not only in pSS group. Another issue is simultaneous with hepatitis C virus (HCV) infection coexistance of clinical and laboratory features of Sjogrens syndrome and accompanying this situation clinical signs of KCS. To sum up symptoms of KCS in primary Sjögren's syndrome and in all patients with DED should be evaluated individually and should take into account the increased risk of infection among these patients.

Keywords: dry eye, infection, Sjögren's syndrome

1. Introduction

Primary Sjögren's syndrome (pSS) is an autoimmune disease in which the symptoms resulting from inflammatory infiltrates in exocrine glands dominate. Frequently, patients complain of a feeling of sand under the eyelids, eye irritation, and red eye caused by a decrease in tear secretion. In pSS, other exocrine glands could be affected—among them: salivary glands, pancreas, vaginal mucous membranes, and glands of gastrointestinal tract or situated in bronchial tree. The patient may complain of dry mouth, dry vagina, and inflammation of the gastric and esophageal reflux. Dry cough may also occur. In the course of pSS interstitial changes in the lungs may occur with a progressive reduction of lung function and a failure of cardiovascular system (in conjunction with the development of right ventricular failure and pulmonary hypertension). Autoimmune inflammatory process may also involve peripheral and central nervous system, including cranial nerves, with symptoms of mixed sensory and motor neuropathy or multiple sclerosis (MS)-like symptoms. In pSS, B lymphocytes (B-cells) play a key role, with their hyperreactivity, leading to the overproduction of autoantibodies. Through the interaction between the cells, stimulation reaches T lymphocytes (T-cells), which are the first to form infiltrates in exocrine glands. The gradual destruction of the exocrine glands by the inflammation and by the autoimmune process causes the above- described symptoms [1].

2. Epidemiology

The epidemiology data of dry eye symptom (DES) reveal that it affects from 5 to 35% of the population. Such discrepancy in the assessment of the frequency of the DES occurrence might be the effect of using different dry eye definitions in each of the studies, as well as the research being performed on different ethnic populations. The data given by the Women's Health Study indicate that Hispanics and Asians display greater predisposition to more severe symptoms of dry eye than Caucasians [2]. The incidence of Sjögren's syndrome, in which DES is a dominant symptom, may also be underestimated. There are no accurate records on the prevalence of this disease, with its milder course prone to be undiagnosed [3,4]. It is estimated that pSS occurs in 0.1–3.0% of the general population. The disease is more common for women (female/male ratio 9:1), affecting mainly individuals between the age of 40 and 60, with the disease most frequently occurring around 50 years of age [5].

3. Outline pathogenesis

The pathogenesis of the disease is not entirely clear and factors responsible for its development are still being sought. It is recognized that environmental or endogenous antigens trigger an inflammatory response in susceptible individuals. Among the environmental factors, several viral infections are considered as primary pSS cause: Epstein-Barr virus (EBV), human T-cell lymphotrophic virus type-1 (HTLV-1), cytomegalovirus (CMV), and hepatitis C virus (HCV) [5–7]. These infections may result in the epithelial barrier damage and the release of autoantigens from the affected epithelial cells. In the case of individual genetic predisposition to pSS, the autoimmune process may develop, involving both mechanisms of innate and adaptive immunity. Genetic factors responsible for the predisposition to pSS development include the presence of HLA-B8, HLA-DW3, HLA-DR3, and DRw52 genes; polymorphism of interferon regulatory factor 5 (IRF 5) gene may also play similar role [1,8]. The release of autoantigens triggers innate immunity through the activation of epithelial (EC) and dendritic cells (DC). DC stimulation promotes interferon I and II pathways; DCs also produce IL-12, which activates natural killer cells (NKCs) and stimulates Th1 cells. Both NKC and Th1 cells secrete interferon gamma (INF-γ), responsible for the tissue damage and stimulating the secretion of B cell activation factor (BAFF). BAFF is produced by T and B cells—both activated by DC; BAFF production is also strongly stimulated by interferon (IFN)-α, released by pDC (plasmocytoid dendritic cells). Moreover, the activation of innate response by Toll-like receptors (TLR-9, TLR-7) additionally increases the secretion of BAFF. This overproduction of BAFF can cause constant stimulation of B cells through different pathways and causes the loss of self-tolerance by T and B cells, overproduction of immunoglobulins, of autoantibodies (predominantly SS-A, SS-B) in particular, and the formation of germinal centres (GC) in the target organs. The affected tissues (especially the salivary glands) display the overexpression of cytokines such as tumor necrosis factor (TNF), lymphotoxin, CXC, and chemokines (ligand 13, 9, 21). This process can lead to the development of lymphoma. The occurrence of primarily marginal zone B-cell lymphoma (MZBCL) has been observed in about 8% of pSS patients—40-fold frequency of the MZBCL in the healthy population [9,10]. The scheme of pathogenesis of pSS is shown on figure1.

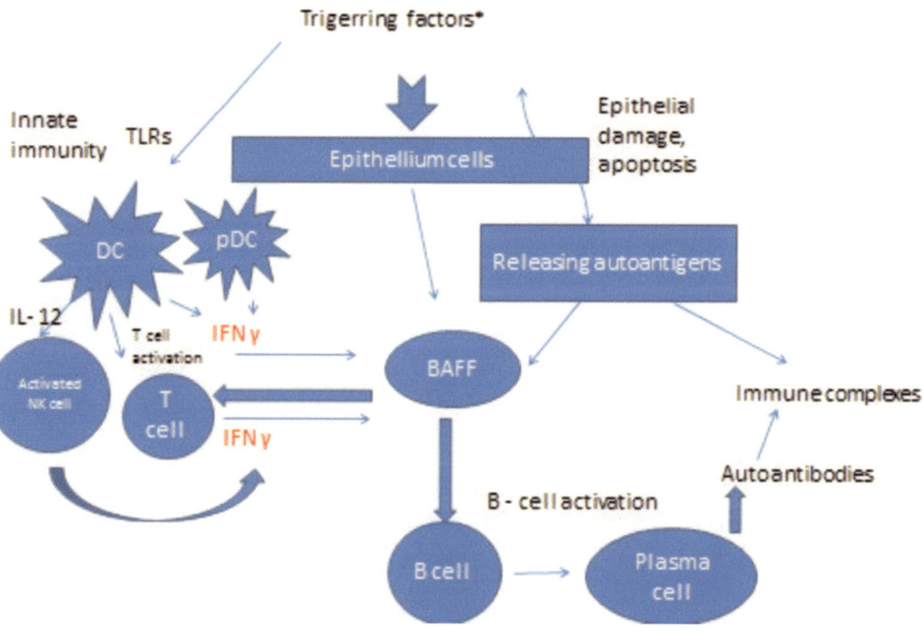

*Triggering factors as viral and bacterial infections, UVA (ultraviolet-A radiation), hormones, genetic predisposition DC-dendritic cell, pDC plasmocytoid DC cell, IFN-γ- interferon gamma, TLRs- Toll-like receptors, IL-12- interleukine 12, TH1-type1 helper cell, BAFF- B cell activating factor, NK-cell natural killer cell

Figure 1. Scheme of pathogenesis [1, 5]

The symptoms of primary Sjögren's syndrome are not homogenous. The autoimmune process involving the epithelium affects many systems and organs, so its manifestations can be very diverse. Symptoms can be divided into two primary groups: common ones, such as dry eyes and mouth, and less frequent symptoms, such as peripheral neuropathy with legs numbness and weakness—with reduced or without reflexes, dysesthesia, feeling of temperature, and vibration. Neurological symptoms may also indicate the seizure of the autonomic nervous system with cardiac arrhythmias or gastrointestinal motility disorder. In the pSS, trigeminal neuralgia and seizure of various nerves ("multiple mononeuropathy") may also occur. The central nervous system can also be involved in pSS therefore myelitis with weakness of limbs and disturbances of urination may occur. Neurological symptoms can also suggest MS, which leads to misdiagnosis. The types of symptoms in pSS are presented in Table 1.

Common symptoms	Less common symptoms/organ involvement
xerophtalmia	intestinal like disease (ILD)
xerostomia	bronchitis
troubles with swallowing	dysphagia, gastrointestinal reflux
dental caries	chronic gastritis
artralgia	symptoms of PBC (primary billary cirrhosis) and AIH
arthritis (non-erosive)	(autoimmune hepatitis)
myalgia	pericarditis
fatigue	pulmonary hypertension
general weakness	celiac-like diseas
weight loss	distal renal tubular acidosis (RTA type 1)
fever	nepritis/glomerulonephritis
Reynaud's phenomenon	chronic renal insufficiency
depression	vasculitis
anxiety	peripheral polyneuropathy,
	cranial neuropathy,
	mononeuritis multiplex
	sensorineural hearing loss
	SM-like syndrome

Table 1. Symptoms of pSS

Keratoconjunctivitis sicca (KCS) is the most frequent cause of complaints from the organ of sight of patients with Sjogren's syndrome, although it can be present in a number of other diseases [11]. KCS is caused by a decreased tear production or increased tear film evaporation. It manifests itself with a feeling of dryness— described as a sandy-gritty eye irritation—burning, stinging, and feeling of tired eyes. In severe cases, the patients suffer from pain, redness, or even decreased vision. The decreased tear production affects the overall reduction of tear secretin as well as limits the aqueous phase of the tears. The causes of DES and complications associated with KCS are presented in Tables 2 and 3.

http://dx.doi.org/10.5772/64243

Primary Sjogren's syndrome may be associated with other autoimmune diseases. Their simultaneous presence can influence both the course and the prognosis of the disease. The most common coexisting diseases are presented in Table 4.

The initial symptoms of an infection in dry eye syndrome—the eye pain, burning, eye redness —can be associated with symptoms of dryness and aseptic KCS, as well as with an incipient infection. However, when the pain and red eye are accompanied by a purulent excretion —a bacterial infection should be suspected. Viral infections primarily cause an eye pain and intense redness. These symptoms may also be associated with general symptoms of infections such as muscle pain, fever, and fatigue. The diagnosis and treatment are determined by the result of the ophthalmological examination.

Keratoconjunctivitis sicca symptoms – conditions and diseases	
Environmental factors as dust, smoke, dry air, aircondition,	Allergic conjunctivitis
Behavior : working at the computer, watching television	Sarcoidosis
long - causing less frequent blinking	Lymphoma
Contact lenses	Graft versus host disease (GvHD)
Age - related dry eye (ARDE)	Autoimmune deficiency (AIDS)
Menopause (low level of estrogens)	Diabetes
Using drugs : antihistamines, β-blockers, diuretics,	Trachoma (cause chlamydia trachomatis)
antispasmodics,	VII cranial nerve damage
diuretics, psychotropic	Meibomian gland dysfunction
Vitami A deficiency	Reflex motor block (central demage of VII cranial nerve)
	Reflex sensory block (trigeminal nerve denervation)
Refractive surgery : laser assisted keratomileusis (LASIK); photorefractive keratoplasty (PRK)	

Table 2. Keratoconjunctivitis sicca —not only symptom of pSS

Eye problems in primary Sjögren's syndrome
discomfort
pain
red eye
conjunctivitis
corneal erosions,
filamentary keratitis,
corneal ulcers
decreased vision

Table 3. Eye complications associated with KCS

The diseases coexisting with p SS
Autoimmune Thyroid Disease (AITD) - Haschimoto disease
Intestinal Lung Disease (ILD)
Primary Billary Cirrhosis (PBC)
Autoimmune hepatitis (AIH)
Cryoglobulinemia
Autoimmune pancreatitis (AIP)
Distal renal tubular acidosis (RTA)
Sclerosis-multiplex like syndrome

Table 4. The diseases coexisting with p SS

4. Risk of eye infections in KCS

The conjunctivitis and changes in the cornea in the pSS are aseptic, yet coexisting infections that may play a part in the development and course of the pSS, KCS in particular. Due to the large differences in estimating the incidence and prevalence of dry eye syndrome (from 5 to 35%) and due to differences in the frequency of recognition of Sjögren's syndrome, it is difficult to accurately estimate the rate of incidence of sicca syndrome associated with eye infections. However, impaired humidification of the eye and related development of KCS undoubtedly significantly increase the risk of bacterial contamination, compared with the normal population.

Among viral infections, EBV plays an important role, which is not limited to the above-mentioned impact on the immune system and lymphocytes. The EBV may be a separate, independent cause of the dry eye syndrome because the infection affects mucosal surfaces and lymphoid tissues. The EBV presence persists in ocular surface epithelia, following primary infection and may cause dacryoadenitis, which leads to abnormal tear secretion [12,13]. Although no direct link between the occurrence of KCS and EBV infection has been established, the influence of EBV on patient's immune status could cause the development of symptoms of dryness. Apart from EBV, other viral infections, which may contribute to the occurrence of KCS and clinical picture of Sjogren's disease, include in particular HCV, human T-cell lymphotropic virus (HTLV), Human (HSV-1), and HIV [7,14]. HCV infection may be responsible for the incidence of ocular symptoms in the course of pSS, such as KCS retinopathy, scleritis, and keratitis. In HSV-1 infection, besides KCS, keratitis, blepharitis, conjunctivitis, uveitis, and retinitis may develop [15]. Viral agents involved in pathogenesis of pSS, EBV in particular, can be simultaneously responsible for causing KCS, conjunctivitis, and reducing resistance of the corneal epithelium.

Although viruses play a significant role in the pathogenesis of pSS, the importance of bacterial co-infections, e.g., *Chlamydia pneumonia* in the course of pSS should not be underestimated [16]. It is known that a tear film has antimicrobial properties, whereas the normal ocular surface contains bacterial flora, including *Staphylococcus epidermidis*, *S. aureus*, and diphteroides (e.g.,

http://dx.doi.org/10.5772/64243

Corynebacterium diphtheriae and *Propionibacterium acnes*). However, in patients with DESs and treated with immunosuppressants, such therapy, along with dryness and cornea damage, results in increased susceptibility to common bacterial infections. In the diagnosis of ocular symptoms, bacterial keratitis should come under consideration. This may more likely be caused by *S. aureus*, *Haemophilus influenzae*, *Streptococcus pneumoniae* and, in the case of use of contact lenses, more often *Pseudomonas aeruginosa*. Hori et al. [17] showed that infections with bacteria resistant to fluoroquinolones (*Staph.* sp. *Staph. aureus*) are more common in patients with dry eye syndrome, although among dry eye patients, regardless of use of punctual plugs or topical steroids, there were no differences in bacteria isolated from conjunctiva.

In the diagnosis of pSS, it must also be considered that some of the commonly known infections, such as HIV, tuberculosis, leprosy, spirochetes, hepatitis A, B, or C, parvovirus B19, Dengue fever, malaria, subacute bacterial endocarditis, and HIV can mimic Sjögren's syndrome with symptoms of eye dryness. Prognosis for the infection occurring in the course of a dry eye in Sjögren's syndrome is more serious compared to the infection cases with no additional risk factors present. This results from the, pre-existing in Sjögren's syndrome, surface damage and use of immunosuppressive therapy in this disease. Therefore, patients with Sjögren's syndrome and a coexisting bacterial infection of the eye belong to a group in which immediate antibiotic therapy should be considered.

5. Cicatrizing conjunctivitis as complication of dry eye disorders

In course of pSS, a slow progressive cicatrizing conjunctivitis (PCC) may also develop with complications such as an impairment of vision (and even blindness), pain, and corneal damage. Cicatrizing is a type of scarring, which can occur as a complication of dry eye accompanied by autoimmune diseases like Sjögren's syndrome or ocular cicatrical pemphigoid. Chronic conjunctival cicatrization (CCC) can also occur as an effect of thermal and chemical burns, postinfectious conjunctivitis, ocular rosacea, atopic keratitis, graft versus host disease, and Stevens-Johnson syndrome (in the latter case prognosis being particularly poor) [18,19]. The presence of cicatrizing conjunctivitis predisposes to microbial keratitis, especially in Sjögren's syndrome. Ormerod et al. [20] described that almost 50% of studied Sjögren's syndrome patients had microbial keratitis as a complication of sterile ulcerations and were subject to recurrent infections. Most common infection in that group was Gram-positive bacteria such as *S. aureus*. It was also noted that patients with conjunctival cicatrization (CC) in the course of Sjögren's syndrome had higher complication rate compared to those in which CC was caused by other factors; such complications included corneal perforation, endophthalmitis, and descementocele. Interestingly, the authors also point out that a long-term therapy with topical corticosteroids and application of bandage contact lenses used in refractive surgery enhanced a risk of microbial keratitis.

Treatment strategies in CC depend on the cause of the underlying disease. In case of microbial keratitis, topical antibiotic use is recommended.

6. Diagnosis criteria of Sjogren's syndrome

Over the years (since 2002), pSS recognition has been based on the criteria set by American-European Consensus Group (AECG) in which both Schirmer's test and tear break-up time (BUT) results are assessed. According to former pSS criteria, the examination of salivary secretory function was assessed by measuring minute salivation and evaluation in sialography. From 2012, the American College of Rheumatology (ACR) has proposed new diagnostic criteria that are presented in Table 5 [21–23].

Sjögren's Syndrome criteria ACR 2012
1. Positive serum anti-SSA/Ro and/or anti-SSB/La or positive rheumatoid factor and ANA titer 1:320
2. Labial salivary gland biopsy exhibiting focal lymphocytic sialadenitis with a focus score 1 focus/4 mm^2
3. Ocular staining score 3 proving keratoconjunctivitis sicca *
Exclusions: Head and neck radiation treatment Active Hepatitis C infection Acquired immunodeficiency syndrome Sarcoidosis Amyloidosis Graft versus host disease (GVHD) IgG4-related disease (IgG4-RD)

*Excluding the patients using daily eye drops for glaucoma and who has had corneal surgery or cosmetic eyelid surgery in the last 5 years

Table 5. Diagnostic criteria of Sjögren's syndrome

It was found that most changes associated with KCS can be demonstrated using the Lissamine green and fluorescein stainings. Both stainings are used for establishing ocular staining score (OSS), determined for each eye separately and used to identify the degree of change in the conjunctiva (Lissamine green) as well as the damage to the cornea (fluorescein) [21]. The slit lamp examination reveals damage to the cornea, but using staining allows for a quantitative and qualitative assessment of these changes. Another test which can be useful in the evaluation of dry eye is a tear osmolality test. However, this test is not included in the criteria for pSS diagnosis [24,25].

The newly proposed criteria also apply to the early stage of diagnosis, when no evidence of the presence of autoantibodies for ribonucleoproteins anti-Ro (SS-A) and anti-La (SS-B) is available. In such a case, the mutual presence of rheumatoid factor (RF) and of antinuclear antibody (ANA, the latter in titer of no less than 1: 320) proves the diagnosis [25].

The important part of establishing pSS diagnosis is confirming the presence of typical changes in histopathology material from minor salivary gland biopsy (MSGB)— mononuclear inflammatory cells form focal infiltrates of more than 50 cells in 4 mm^2 of glandular section. The so-called focus score (FS) is based on the assessment of number of such changes in the tested material. The presence of one or more foci is considered as a positive result. Primary Sjogren's syndrome may be accompanied by other than SS-A, SS-B, or RF autoantibodies [26,27]. Most common pSS-specific antibodies, also associated with other autoimmune diseases, are presented in Table 6.

Autoantibodies in pSS
diagnostic hallmark:
Anti SS-A (Ro)
Anti-SS-B (La)
Autoantibodies in pSS and other autoimmune diseases:
Antinuclear antibodies (ANAs)
Rheumatoid factors (RF)
Anti-centromere antibodies (ACA) (systemic sclerosis)
Anti-mitochondrial antibodies (AMA) - Primary biliary cirrhosis
Anti-cyclic citrullinated peptide antibodies (anti-CCP)
anti-smooth muscle antibodies (ASMA) Autoimmune hepatitis
dsDNA (systemic lupus erythematosus)
Anti- thyreoglobulin (anti TG) – autoimmune thyroiditis
Anti-thyroid peroxidase (anti-TPO)- autoimmune thyroiditis
Novel autoantibodies:
Anti-M3R antibodies
Anti- β fodrin
Anti - protein 1 (SP-1),
Anti - carbonic anhydrase 6 (CA6)
Anti-parotid secretory protein (PSP)

Table 6. Autoantibodies in pSS

Several laboratory tests prove helpful in the diagnosis of pSS, although they do not constitute a part of the present diagnostic pSS criteria. In particular, the deviations in the composition of blood cells and proteins occur and the increased erythrocyte sedimentation rate (ESR) with normal or low concentrations of CRP (a similar situation may exist in multiple myeloma) may be present. Laboratory findings in pSS are presented in Table 7.

Laboratory findings in pSS
Elevated erythrocyte sedimentation rate (ESR),
leucopenia,
anemia
low platelet count
Hypergammaglobulinemia (polyclonal),
ANAs, RF, anti-Ro/SS-A, anti-B/SSB,
decreased level of complement component C4

Table 7. Laboratory findings in pSS

Llissamine green (conjunctiva)		Fluoresceine (cornea)	
grade	dots	grade	dots
0	0-9	0	0
1	10-32	1	1-5
2	33- 100	2	6- 30
3	> 100	3	> 30

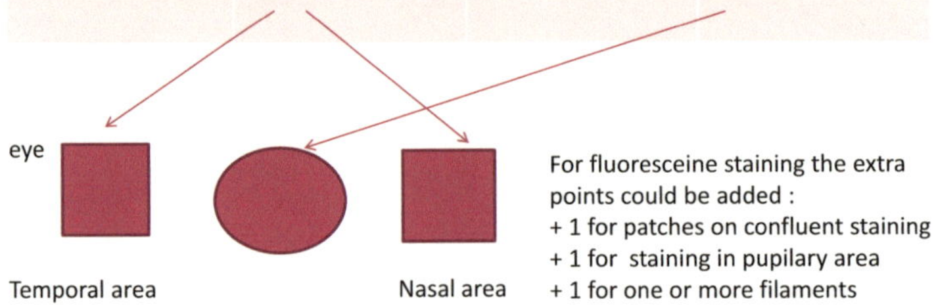

Figure 2. Sicca ocular staining score [25]

7. Prognosis

The emergence of pSS carries an increased risk (by 40 times – comparing to the normal population) of lymphoma development. This imposes necessity of regular monitoring and assessment in pSS of factors/markers determining patient's total capacity for developing lymphoma, including the emergence of cryoglobulins, rheumatoid factor (if previously not present) or of monoclonal proteins, chronic enlargement of the salivary glands, or persistent presence of general symptoms, such as weight loss, fever, and lymphadenopathy.

7.1. Eye examinations for the diagnosis of KCS and pSS

The ophthalmic examination includes first of all a well-known Schirmer's test used to evaluate the extent of decrease in the tear secretion.

In the case of significant intensity of dry eye syndrome, the damage to the cornea can be visualized by applying lissamine green and fluorescein staining [28]. This scoring system has been proposed for the evaluation of KCS in Sjögren's syndrome, but applies in general to the changes in the course of dry eye.

The scoring rules are illustrated in Figure 2, and photographs of eye examination in Figures 3 and 4.

The maximum score for each eye is 12. Scoring more than 3 and higher indicates KCS.

The previous AECG pSS diagnosis criteria consisted, in addition to the Schirmer's test, in other tests confirming the presence of KCS and lacrimation disorder, with Bengal rose staining among the most frequently used. This test allows for the assessment of scaly, dead cells of the corneal epithelium, and conjunctiva as well as mucus particles (filaments) fixed to the corneal

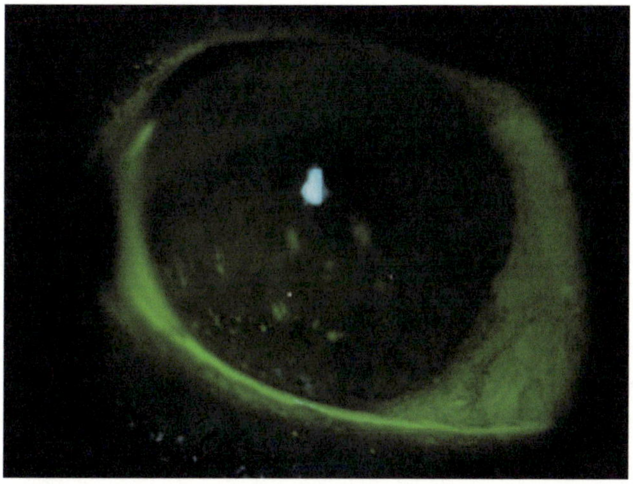

Figure 3. Fluorescein staining

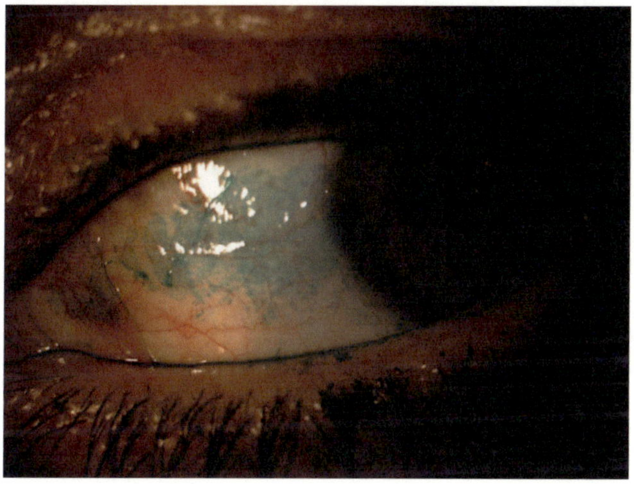

Figure 4. Lissamine green staining

surface, associated with the dry eye syndrome. The results of rose Bengal staining, however, are dose-dependent and cause phototoxicity. The lissamine green dye is less irritating and thus considered better for such use. The quality and quantity of the tear film can be evaluated using tear film break up time (T-BUT)—assessing the time interval between the last complete blink and the first appearance of a dry spot or of disruption of the tear film, observed in the slit lamp. The extension of this test uses fluorescein (F-BUT) staining. The diagnosis of DES is established with BUT result ≤5 seconds. The limitations of this test are eye irritation and increased blink after fluorescein application as well as difficulty in meeting the condition that the patient can blink freely [28].

7.2. Own research

In our study, 30 patients—22 females (73%), 8 males (27%) in mean age of 52 years (from 22 to 85)—diagnosed with pSS revealed stronger correlation of the Schirmer's test results with FS than with OSS. The correlation coefficient of OSS with ANA, anti–SS-A, RF was higher than that of Schirmer's test with anti–SS-A and RF. OSS correlated negatively with Schirmer's test results (r= −0.54; p=0.007). There were no differences between female and male subjects in the Schirmer's test, a group of male patients presented more pronounced symptoms of ocular dryness in the evaluation of staining scores. Our results suggest that the Schirmer's test reflects the intensity of ocular gland infiltration by inflammatory cells, whereas immunostaining proposed in the new Sjögren's syndrome criteria is more closely associated with the immunoactivity and autoantibodies production. It is obvious that the observed correlation requires further support and analysis of research performed on a more numerous group of patients.

7.2.1. Statistical analysis

Correlation analyses were performed with the Spearman correlation coefficient (because of the non-normal distribution of variables). The study was approved by the Bioethics Commission of the Institute of Rheumatology; the subjects have signed written informed consent statements. The study was supported by National Science Center (Narodowe Centrum Nauki) —grant no. 2012/05/N/NZ5/02838. The correlations are shown in Table 8.

Correlations	Correlation coefficient (Spearman test) N=30
OSS mean– SS-A	0,17
OSS mean– SS- B	0,00
OSS mean – FS	0,13
OSS mean – RF	0,04
OSS mean – ANA	-0,16
Schirmer's test mean – SS-A	-0,10
Schirmer's test mean – SS-B	0,14
Schirmer's test mean – FS	0,07
Schirmer's test mean – RF	0,20
test Schirmera średnia – ppj	-0,01
SA-A – SS-B	0,56
OSS mean – Schirmer's test mean	-0,54
Ro – FS	0,04
Ro – RF	0,20
Ro – ppj	0,25
La – FS	0,07
La – RF	0,20
La – ppj	0,27

Table 8. Correlations in patients group with pSS

The data were presented at the 3rd International Congress on Controversies in Rheumatology and Autoimmunity in 2014 [29]. Toker et al. [30] also studied the presence of anti–SS/A and anti–SS/B antibodies in tears and serum as well as assessed the correlations between subjective and objective clinical score of dry eye (then performed Schirmer's test, TBUT test, and rose Bengal staining). This study demonstrated that serum titer of anti-Ro/SSA and anti-La/SSB correlated positively with DESs and negatively with tear production.

7.3. Treatment of pSS

1. Systemic treatment of Sjogren's syndrome

The therapy of autoimmune diseases, such as pSS, is based on the elimination of inflammation and inhibition of stimulation of the immune system. Initially, immunosuppressant drugs, such as corticosteroids, methotrexate, cyclosporine A, and azathioprine are applied. For years, the effectiveness and relevance of applying antimalaria drugs for the treatment of pSS have been debated [31–33]. A number of studies confirm beneficial effects of this drug on the symptoms of dryness and the reduction of BAFF in patients with pSS without significant internal organ involvement [32–34]. In severe cases with life threatening organ involvement, the use of cyclophosphamide, infusions of immunoglobulins, and plasmapheresis are considered necessary.

In the case of renal tubular acidosis, sodium and/or potassium are administered. Considering the role of B cells in pSS, monoclonal anti-CD20 (rituximab RTX) antibodies seem to be a favorable option for therapy. RTX has already shown efficacy in the treatment of rheumatoid arthritis, SLE, and vasculitis [35–37]. The full effectiveness of other biologic drugs causing the depletion of B cells—such as Belimumab (BLyS/BAFF inhibitor) and epratuzumab (humanized anti-CD22 monoclonal antibody)—has not yet been confirmed in pSS treatment [38]. The purpose of the therapy could also be the inhibition of interferon alpha and gamma (IFN-α and IFN-γ) involved in the stimulation of B cells, but this course of therapy requires further study.

Currently, the use of mesenchymal stem cell (MSC) transplantation as a method of treatment of various autoimmune diseases, including Sjogren's syndrome, is also being contemplated [39].

2. Topical treatment—the fight against dryness

Apart from the systemic treatment, no less important for pSS patients is local treatment and alleviation of dryness symptoms. Firstly, in the case of dry eye, the influence of exacerbating factors, such as dryness, dust, long hours of working with computer, and smoking, should be limited. It is recommended to use artificial tears during the day and lubricant ointment at night. Agents used as preservatives in medical drops, even those in moisturizers- among them: benzalkonium chloride (BAK) and disodium (EDTA) pose another problem [40]. The use of over-the-counter (OTC) drops with a higher dose of preservatives increases the symptoms of dryness [41].

The wide array of medications is being used in topical treatment: eye lubricants and moisturizers, such as drops, gels, ointments containing tear substitutes, oils and petrolatum, acrylic acid, hyaluronic acid, glycerin, erythritol, levocarnitine, hydroxymethylcellose, carboxymethylcelulose, or glycol. The preparations without preservatives that replace tears include, e.g., Refresh (Allergan), TheraTears, Soothe (Bausch + Lomb), and System (Alcon) [41].

Ocular lubricants and moisturizers are designed to supplement the shortage of tears, osmolarity, and to improve tear film stability and act protectively. A patient with severe DES both in the course of PSS and from other causes, however, should consult the use of these substances with an ophthalmologist. Increasing the amount of tears can be achieved by permanent occluding of nasolacrimal channel and by the use of biological tear substitutes, namely a drop of the patient's own serum. The inflammatory process in the course KCS also requires anti-inflammatory therapy with cyclosporine drops and topical glucocorticoids. Research is being conducted on the use of pimecrolimus and tacrolimus as immunomodulatory drugs in drops. Also drugs stimulating tear secretion with cholinergic agonists are being used and two of them, namely pilocarpine and cevimeline, are used widely. Currently, studies are being carried out on other stimulants, among others diquafosol (P2Y2 receptor agonist) and rebamipide [42,43].

Tetracyclines (minocycline, tetracycline) might also be considered as important drugs for pSS therapy, showing both antibacterial and immunomodulating effect. They have greater than just antimicrobial effect on inflammation by inhibiting the proinflammatory cytokines as TNF or interleukin-1 (IL-1) and also inhibiting angiogenesis. They have been applied to treat eye infections, ocular and skin manifestations of acne rosacea and are used in the case of meibomian gland dysfunction [44]. In the case of complications of bacterial infection in the course of KCS, typical antibiotics covering the activities of most common pathogens are being used. These include aminoglycosides (e.g., Tobramycin), macrolides, fluoroquinolones, sodium sulfacetamide, or trimethoprim/polymyxin. While wearing contact lenses is as a possible cause of dry eye, in the treatment of DES contact lenses made of special materials such as silicone rubber and highly oxygen permeable materials may protect the eye from drying [45,46].

The surgical treatment, including placement of punctual plugs (collagen or silicone) and cauterization of the puncta, is used in cases of severe corneal injuries and at a risk of a loss of vision. The transplantation of minor salivary glands is an interesting and promising method, but so far with limited use as a therapeutic option [47]. The salivary glands are transplanted as a complex graft to the posterior lamella of the eyelids to increase an ocular surface lubrication and reduce a discomfort in dry eyes.

Frequent blinking is also important for the prophylaxis and complementary action treatment for symptoms of dry eye; avoiding situations that increase the evaporation of the tear film (e.g. wind, air conditioning, and smoking) is recommended as well. The patients with pSS and symptoms of dry eye should be controlled both by a rheumatologist and an ophthalmologist. Routine check of a dry eye should take place at least once every 3 months. However ophthalmologic monitoring frequency will depend on the severity of DESs and the presence of dry eye complications, such as infections. In the latter case, the control should be performed every few days until the infection is cured. The aim of the topical therapy is to eliminate symptoms of dryness and to directly protect mucous membranes. The systemic treatment is directed at achieving a remission—the inhibition of the disease progress, changes in internal organs, and inflammation and infiltration of exocrine glands.

8. Summary

The Sjögren's syndrome is one of the most common rheumatic diseases with predominant symptoms of dryness, particularly of the eye. Therefore, the knowledge on dry eye disease or KCS symptoms is essential not only for ophthalmologic but also for rheumatologic practice. The above section certainly does not exhaust the problem of Sjögren's syndrome, its intricate and still uncertain pathogenesis and a differentiated clinical picture. The author's intention was primarily to draw attention to the problem of DESs and associated complications, including infections.

Author details

Maria Maślińska* and Brygida Kwiatkowska

*Address all correspondence to: maslinskam@gmail.com

Early Arthritis Clinic, National Institute of Geriatrics, Rheumatology and Rehabilitation the name of Prof. Eleonora Reicher, Warsaw, Poland

References

[1] Youinou P, Pers JO. Disturbance of cytokine networks in Sjögren's syndrome. Arthritis Res Ther. 2011;13:227.

[2] McCarty CA, Bansal AK, Livingston PM, Stanislavsky YL, Taylor HR. The epidemiology of dry eye in Melbourne, Australia. Ophthalmology. 1998;105(6):1114–9.

[3] Viso E, Rodriguez-Ares MT, Gude F. Prevalence of and associated factors for dry eye in a Spanish adult population (the Salnes Eye Study). Ophthalmic Epidemiol. 2009;16(1):15–21. doi: 10.1080/09286580802228509.

[4] Lee AJ, Lee J, Saw SM, Gazzard G, Koh D, Widjaja D, Tan DT. Prevalence and risk factors associated with dry eye symptoms: a population based study in Indonesia. Br J Ophthalmol. 2002;86(12):1347–51.

[5] Maślińska M, Przygodzka M, Kwiatkowska B, Sikorska-Siudek K Sjögren's syndrome: still not fully understood disease Rheumatol Int. 2015 ;35:233–41 DOI 10.1007/s00296-014-3072-5

[6] Slobod KS, Sandlund JT, Spiegel PH et al. Molecular evidence of ocular Epstein-Barr virus infection. Clin Infect Dis. 2000;31(1):184–8.

[7] Pinheiro SR, Martins-Filho OA, Ribas JG, Catalan-Soares BC, Proietti FA, Namen-Lopes S, et al. Immunologic markers, uveitis, and keratoconjunctivitis sicca associat-

ed with human T-cell lymphotropic virus type 1. Am J Ophthalmol. 2006;142(5):811–5.

[8] Miceli-Richard C, Comets E, Loiseau P, Puechal X, Hachulla E, Mariette X. Association of an IRF5 gene functional polymorphism with Sjögren's syndrome. Arthritis Rheum. 2007;56(12):3989–94.

[9] Huang YF, Cheng Q, Jiang CM, et al. The immune factors involved in the pathogenesis, diagnosis, and treatment of Sjogren's syndrome. Clin Dev Immunol. Vol. 2013(2013). Article ID 160491. doi: 10.1155/2013/160491

[10] Baimpa E, Dahabreh IJ, Voulgarelis M, Moutsopoulos HM. Hematologic manifestations and predictors of lymphoma development in primary Sjögren syndrome: clinical and pathophysiologic aspects. Medicine (Baltimore) 2009; 88(5):284–293.

[11] Lemp MA. Report of the National Eye Institute/Industry Workshop on Clinical Trials in Dry Eyes. CLAO J. 1995;21(4):221–32.

[12] Merayo-Lloves J, Baltatzis S, Foster CS. Epstein-Barr virus dacryoadenitis resulting in keratoconjunctivitis sicca in a child. Am J Ophthalmol. 2001;132(6):922–3.

[13] Rhem MN, Wilhelmus KR, Jones DB. Epstein-Barr virus dacryoadenitis. Am J Ophthalmol. 2000;129(3):372–5.

[14] Bekele S, Gelaw Y, Tessema F. Ocular manifestation of HIV/AIDS and correlation with CD4+ cells count among adult HIV/AIDS patients in Jimma town, Ethiopia: a cross sectional study. BMC Ophthalmol. 2013;27;13:20. doi: 10.1186/1471-2415-13-20.

[15] Alves M, Angerami RN, Rocha EM. Dry eye disease caused by viral infection: review. Arq Bras Oftalmol. 2013;76(2):129–32.

[16] Krásny J, Hrubá D, Netuková M. The role of Chlamydia pneumoniae in the etiology of keratoconjunctivitis sicca (KCS). Recent Pat Inflamm Allergy Drug Discov. 2014;8(3):216–22.

[17] Hori Y1, Maeda N, Sakamoto M, Koh S, Inoue T, Tano Y. Bacteriologic profile of the conjunctiva in the patients with dry eye. Am J Ophthalmol. 2008 Nov;146(5):729-34. doi: 10.1016/j.ajo.2008.06.003. Epub 2008 Jul 30.

[18] Faraj HG, Hoang-Xuan T. Chronic cicatrizing conjunctivitis. Curr Opin Ophthalmol. 2001;12(4):250–7.

[19] Rashida S, Danaa M. Cicatrizing and autoimmune diseases. Chem Immunol Allergy. Basel, Karger, 2007 (92):195–202.

[20] Ormerod LD, Fong LP, Foster CS. Corneal infection in mucosal Scarring Disorders and Sjogren's syndrome. Am J Ophthalmology 1988;105:512–18.

[21] Shiboski SC, Shiboski CH, Criswell L, et al. American College of Rheumatology classification criteria for Sjögren's syndrome: a data-driven, expert consensus approach

in the Sjögren's International Collaborative Clinical Alliance cohort. Arthritis Care Res (Hoboken) 2012;64(4):475–87.

[22] Vitali C, Bootsma H, Bowman SJ, et al. Classification criteria for Sjögren's syndrome: we actually need to definitively resolve the long debate on the issue. Ann Rheum Dis. 2013;72:476–78.

[23] Rasmussen A, Ice JA, Li H, et al. Comparison of the American-European Consensus Group Sjögren's syndrome classification criteria to newly proposed American College of Rheumatology criteria in a large, carefully characterized sicca cohort. Ann Rheum Dis 2014;73(1): 31- 8. doi:10.1136/annrheumdis-2013-203845

[24] Tomlinson A. 2007. DEWS Report, Ocular Surface April 2007 Vol 5 No 2.

[25] Rose-Nussbaumer J, Lietman TM, Shiboski CH, et al. Sjögren's International Collaborative Clinical Alliance Research Groups. Inter-grader Agreement of the Ocular Staining Score in the Sjögren's International Clinical Collaborative Alliance (SICCA) registry. Am J Ophthalmol. 2015 ; 21. pii: S0002-9394(15)00515-2. doi: 10.1016/j.ajo. 2015.08.021. [Epub ahead of print].

[26] Kyriakidis NC, Kapsogeorgou EK, Tzioufas AG. A comprehensive review of autoantibodies in primary Sjogren's syndrome: clinical phenotypes and regulatory mechanisms. J Autoimmun 2003; 51C:67–74.

[27] Shen L, Suresh L, Lindemann M, et al. Novel autoantibodies in Sjogren's syndrome. Clin Immunol 2012;145(3):251–255.

[28] Whitcher JP, Shiboski CH, Shiboski SC, et al. Sjögren's International Collaborative Clinical Alliance Research Groups. A simplified quantitative method for assessing keratoconjunctivitis sicca from the Sjögren's syndrome International Registry. Am J Ophthalmol. 2010;149(3):405–15. doi: 10.1016/j.ajo.2009.09.013. Epub 2009 Dec 29.

[29] Maślińska M. Szymczak – Mikołowska. The degree of correlation between ocular tests, autoantibodies presence and salivary gland inflammatory infiltration in primary Sjögren's syndrome. Index No.260 3rd International Congress on Controversies in Rheumatology and Autoimmunity in 2014.

[30] Toker E, Yavuz S, Direskeneli H.Anti-Ro/SSA and anti-La/SSB autoantibodies in the tear fluid of patients with Sjögren's syndrome. Br J Ophthalmol. 2004;88:384–87.

[31] Bron JB, Abelson BM, Ousler G, et al. Methodologies to diagnose and monitor dry eye disease: Report of the Diagnostic Methodology Subcommittee of the International Dry Eye Workshop. Ocul Surf. 2007;5(2):108–52.

[32] Mumcu G, Biçakçigil M, Yilmaz N, Ozay H, Karaçayli U, Cimilli H, Yavuz S. Salivary and serum B-cell activating factor (BAFF) levels after hydroxychloroquine treatment in primary Sjögren's syndrome. Oral Health Prev Dent. 2013;11(3):229–34. doi: 10.3290/j.ohpd.a30172.

[33] Yavuz S1, Asfuroğlu E, Bicakcigil M, Toker E. Hydroxychloroquine improves dry eye symptoms of patients with primary Sjogren's syndrome. Rheumatol Int. 2011;31(8):1045–9. doi: 10.1007/s00296-010-1415-4. Epub 2010 Mar 23.

[34] Rihl M1, Ulbricht K, Schmidt RE, Witte T. Treatment of sicca symptoms with hydroxychloroquine in patients with Sjogren's syndrome. Rheumatology (Oxford). 2009;48(7): 796–9. doi: 10.1093/rheumatology/kep104. Epub 2009 May 11.

[35] Chen S, Liu Y, Shi G. Anti-CD20 antibody in primary Sjögren's syndrome management. Curr Pharm Biotechnol. 2014;15(6):535–41.

[36] St Clair EW, Levesque MC, Prak ET, Vivino FB, Alappatt CJ, Spychala ME, Wedgwood J, McNamara J, Moser Sivils KL, Fisher L, Cohen P. Autoimmunity Centers of Excellence. Rituximab therapy for primary Sjögren's syndrome: an open-label clinical trial and mechanistic analysis. Arthritis Rheum. 2013;65(4):1097–106. doi: 10.1002/art.37850.

[37] Vossenkämper A, Lutalo PM, Spencer J Translational Mini-Review Series on B cell subsets in disease. Transitional B cells in systemic lupus erythematosus and Sjögren's syndrome: clinical implications and effects of B cell-targeted therapies. Clin Exp Immunol. 2012; 167(1):7–14.

[38] Steinfeld SD, Tant L, Burmester GR et al. Epratuzumab (humanised anti-CD22 antibody) in primary Sjögren's syndrome: an open-label phase I/II study. Arthritis Res Ther. 2006;8(4):R129.

[39] Xu J, Wang D, Liu D, Fan Z, et al. Allogeneic mesenchymal stem cell treatment alleviates experimental and clinical Sjögren syndrome. Blood 2012;120(15):3142–51.

[40] Sarkar J, Chaudhary, Namavari A, et al. Corneal neurotoxicity due to topical benzalkonium chloride. Invest Ophthalmol Vis Sci. 2012;53(4):1792–802.

[41] Stephenson M. OTC Drops: Telling the Tears Apart. When choosing an over-the-counter artificial tear for your dry-eye patient, consider severity of disease and form of dry eye. Rev Ophtalmol. 2012; 19 (10):31-37. www.reviewofophthalmology.com/content/i/2133/c/36940/

[42] Keating GM. Diquafosol ophthalmic solution 3 %: a review of its use in dry eye. Drugs. 2015;75(8):911–22. doi: 10.1007/s40265-015-0409-7.

[43] Ueda K, Matsumiya W, Otsuka K, Maeda Y, Nagai T, Nakamura M. Effectiveness and relevant factors of 2% rebamipide ophthalmic suspension treatment in dry eye. BMC Ophthalmol. 2015;15:58. doi: 10.1186/s12886-015-0040-0.

[44] Kwiatkowska B, Maslinska M, Przygodzka M, Dmowska-Chalaba J, Dabrowska J, Sikorska-Siudek K. Immune system as a new therapeutic target for antibiotics. Adv Biosci Biotechnol. 2013;4:91–101.

[45] Bacon AS, Astin C, Dart JK. Silicone rubber contact lenses for the compromised cornea. Cornea. 1994;13(5):422–8.

[46] Romero-Rangel T, Stavrou P, Cotter J, Rosenthal P, Baltatzis S, Foster CS. Gas-permeable scleral contact lens therapy in ocular surface disease. Am J Ophthalmol. 2000;130(1):25–32.

[47] Geerling G, Raus P, Murube J. Minor salivary gland transplantation. Dev Ophthalmol. 2008;41:243–54. doi: 10.1159/000131093.